Caring for Children With Sickle Cell Disease

A Mother's Perspective

I0225451

Olana's World

https://agnesnsofwa.com.au/

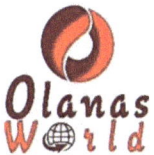

Olanas World

ISBN: 978-0-6454134-9-6

CONTENTS

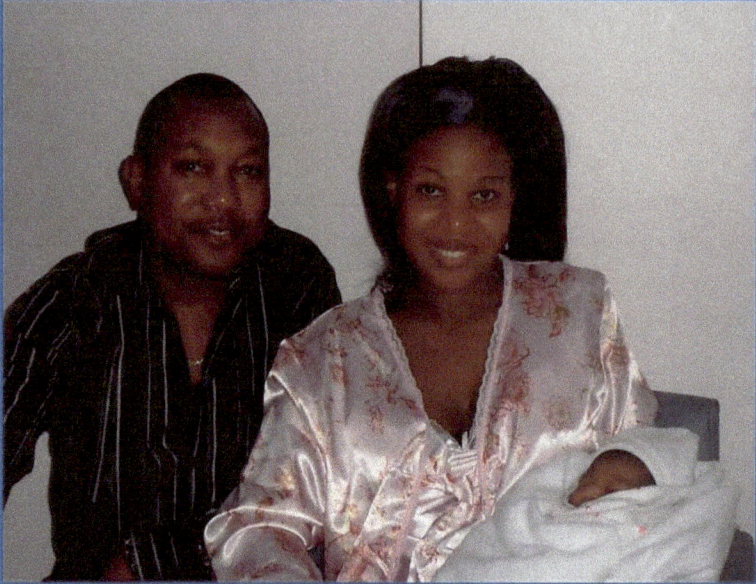

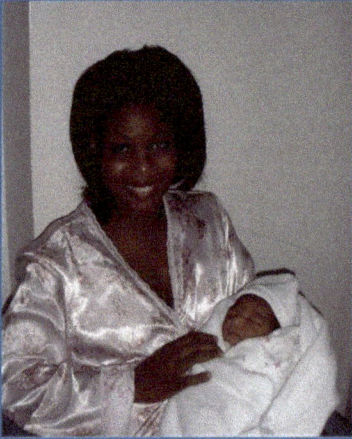

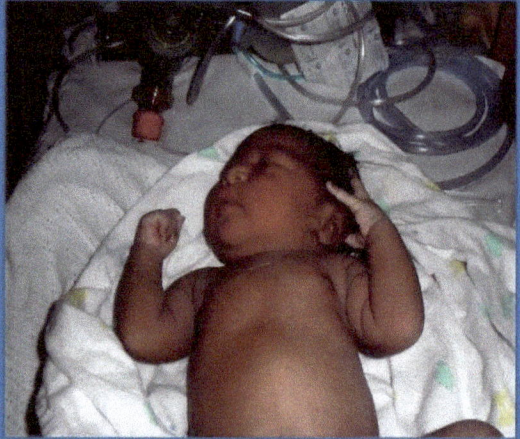

Foreword

"Your child has sickle cell." Five impactful words that change everything for the family, particularly the mother on the receiving end. This book gives the reader a front row seat on this journey, from the lowest of lows to the small and monumental wins.

Despite sickle cell disease (SCD) being the first genetic disease to be examined at the molecular level, it has been widely ignored by medical researchers, resulting in limited treatment options and resources. This is a devastating disease that can result in organ damage and early mortality. It is most commonly known for the severe pain crisis it causes, whih is outwardly invisible to others. As a result, individuals who suffer from this condition (called sickle cell warriors) are not treated with the care and compassion they deserve because of stigma and stereotypes; this is one of the most heartbreaking experiences faced by sickle cell warriors. Even when in the care of healthcare professionals, ensuring that individuals consistently get the recommended care and pain medications rests heavily upon the family/advocates.

Typically, mothers are the family at the bedside, spending countless nights in hospitals with their children. I was connected to Agnes in 2022 by a friend and colleague primarily because of our shared experience of having a child with sickle cell disease. Even over the few years I have known her, she continues to make strides for the sickle cell community in Australia. She took her despair and turned it into an organisation for hope; her passion and zeal for improved care for individuals with this disease go well beyond her daughter. Clearly, she will not rest until sickle cell care is available for all impacted in Australia and beyond. Her journey to becoming a nurse is fascinating and incredible. As the founder of the Australia Sickle Cell Advocacy Inc., she has led numerous advocacy efforts on behalf of families and individuals living with this condition, one of the most impactful being the adoption of universal newborn screening for sickle cell in the Australian Health system in September 2024. She has worked with healthcare professionals, schools, employers, and policy makers to ensure individuals with SCD are heard, seen, and their needs accommodated to enable them to achieve their full potential.

She shines a light on the mother or caregivers' journey and shares valuable information on advocacy, clear communication, self-care, fears, trials, tribulations, and the vulnerabilities faced. The chapter on the curative therapy journey for her family is especially hopeful for others. In summary, this book does not provide shortcuts nor sugarcoat the burden that having a family member with sickle cell disease is, and yet it provides a calming strength and hope for others who may find themselves on a similar journey.

What started as a way to help her daughter has transformed and positively impacted the lives of many in Australia and beyond!

Mamle Anim, MD FACP

August 2025

From Pain to Purpose: When a mother becomes a sickle cell advocate

A Personal Thanks

To my daughter P: your bravery is my inspiration. Every day you teach me that courage is not the absence of fear, but the determination to act despite it. Thank you for allowing me to be your mum and for your help to highlight this condition. Love you so much, kiddo.

To our hero, Ms. B, thank you for your selfless act of giving your sister a second chance at life. You never questioned, you never doubted; you knew how your pelvis would be drilled to harvest the marrow, but did you ever say you would not go through with it? You are our hero, thank you, kiddo, love you so much.

To my husband Preston: thank you for your steady hand and your shared hope. This path has tested us both, and you never let me walk it alone.

To Ms. Sanda and Mr. Kuka, you have been the best elder siblings any parent could ask for. You were forced to grow up faster than any of your peers. With numerous hospital visits, you learnt how to care for yourselves and your sisters. I love you guys so much. Thank you for everything you continue to do.

To our family, friends, and community: thank you for holding space for our grief and celebrating our joy. Your warmth has been the scaffolding of our resilience.

To the healthcare teams: we know you walk a challenging path, too. To those who learned, listened, and loved when we felt unseen, thank you.

To every parent who's ever waited by a hospital bed, afraid, may you feel less alone. May this book be a light in the dark and a companion in your journey.

When your child is diagnosed with sickle cell disease, your world changes overnight.

I know this because I have personally experienced it.

Suddenly, you're no longer just a mother; you become a nurse, researcher, counsellor, and fierce protector.

Every hospital visit, every pain crisis, every sleepless night lights a fire inside you.

That fire? It often turns into advocacy. I have seen a lot of mothers like me turn that fire into finding solutions.

Mothers become advocates, not because we choose to, but because we must. No matter how difficult that road looks or what others think, we endure the journey.

We raise awareness, fight for better healthcare access, advocate for policy change, and support other families navigating the same challenging path.

We understand the system, the gaps, and most importantly, the stakes.

Advocacy becomes a form of healing.

It gives our children a voice.

It guides others through the unknown.

And it challenges silence with action.

Behind every sickle cell policy, campaign, or community event, there's likely a mother like me who refused to stay quiet.

Introduction:
From Pain to Possibility

There is a love which transcends description, a powerful, unstoppable force of love which dwells from the very core of a parent's being when their child is in pain. It is the kind of love that outstrips fatigue, that outstrips fear, that draws strength from the most unlikely places. This is not a gentle love, it's the love of a warrior, keen, constant, and inexorable. It's the kind of love that influenced every step of my path as a mom to a child with sickle cell disease (SCD), a lifelong inherited blood disorder I'd hardly known existed before it became such a part of our lives.

I was unprepared when my daughter was diagnosed. Aside from vague memories of hearing about it in high school from my peers who were affected, I had no prior knowledge of SCD. I also didn't grasp the life-changing effects, the endless doctor visits, the midnight fevers, the frantic trips to the emergency room, the devastating unpredictability of pain crises, and the slow emotional toll on both the patient and the family. I didn't realise it would alter my life forever the moment she was diagnosed, but it did. And this book tells the story of that transformation, from the early days of chaos and helplessness, through the years of confusion and fear that followed, to the point when my daughter underwent a bone marrow transplant that saved her life and gave her another chance.

I'm no scientist, and I'm certainly no doctor; I am a mother. I am a witness to the suffering, a guardian in the hospital corridors, a voice on behalf of my child when she could not speak, a candle in the dark, and a hug when her body betrayed her in ways no child should ever have to endure. I've had to figure out how to give her medications, spot early signs of infection, make sense of lab results, and fiercely advocate for her needs. But none of that was accompanied by a manual. I learned while living it, while surviving it, and while loving my child through every single moment.

This is not only a story about my daughter's illness, but also about the lived reality of parenting a child with a chronic condition that seeps into every crevice of life. Sickle cell disease is relentless; it is physical, yes, but it is also psychological, social, academic, familial, and, yes, religious. There were times when we felt truly and achingly alone because so few people in our orbit knew what we were going through. Most of the world continued as usual, while our lives centred on easing her pain, following a schedule for hydration, seeking transfusions, and waiting for news that could alter everything.

Sickle cell disease is often discussed in the sterile, clinical language of medical textbooks. It's a genetic condition in which red blood cells, which are supposed to be round and pliable, instead become rigid and crescent-shaped. These deformed cells become lodged in blood vessels, obstructing blood circulation and leading to episodes of excruciating pain, organ damage, and other life-threatening conditions. But no textbook description, no matter how horrific, can convey what it's like to watch your child writhing in pain as you stand there helpless to stop it. No chart or pie graph can capture the fear of seeing a fever spike in the middle of the night or the helplessness of watching your own child fall behind at school because she missed too many days lying in bed.

For years, we were told there was no cure, only management. Pain crises could be treated. Complications could be monitored. We were instructed to be vigilant, to steer clear of triggers like dehydration or going out in the cold, to keep her stress as low as possible (as if stress could be eliminated from your life when you were living with a chronic illness). We just had to make it through one catastrophe after another, holding our breath between crises, hoping for a couple of good weeks of peace. We became accustomed to living on the edge.

And then there was the hope for a cure, a bone marrow transplant. It was a hard decision for us. The process itself is gruelling, dangerous, and emotionally excruciating. But we understood that if we could give our daughter a life with less pain, a life with less time in hospitals, less time on medication, and more freedom, we had to try. That chapter of our story, too, is one I'll be recounting in this book, including all the specifics, struggles, and small miracles in between.

This book is organised into chapters reflecting various seasons in our journey. From the denial with which many families cope when a child is diagnosed and in the vulnerable early years of childhood, through the turbulent emotions of adolescence, to confronting a decision of incredible magnitude, to transplant or to forever remain as they are, each stage has its own lessons, heartbreaks, and hopes too large for words. The days we thought we might not go on. And there were moments when we were shocked by how much we could tolerate. There were losses, but there were also wins. Amid it all, though, there was love, not the kind of love that shies away from suffering.

For so many reasons, I found myself needing to write this book. As they say, I wrote it first and foremost for the parents who are scared and confused, as I once was. I want you to remember, you are not alone. Your pain, your exhaustion, your fierce love, they're visible and palpable. I wrote it for those children who suffer from SCD; for them to know that their stories are essential. They deserve to be acknowledged. I wrote it for larger families, teachers, friends, and caregivers who want to help someone with SCD but don't always know how. I wrote it to the doctors and nurses, so that they knew what it feels like to be on the other side of the chart. I wrote it to educate communities about a disease that affects millions worldwide but is often misunderstood and underfunded.

The book is also a homage to the resilience of children who endure pain with a grace that belies their years. It's a love letter to the endurance of families who come together for one another. And it's a celebration of hope of how far medical science has come and of how one bone marrow donor gifted my daughter with everything.

But let's say you are the one holding this book, whatever role you play, it may be as a parent, caregiver, grandparent, healthcare provider, or someone seeking to learn more. I thank you. Thank you for joining us for a stroll. Thank you for taking us to yours. I post it not because it is unique, but because it is just one among tens of thousands of untold stories. There is a family like mine behind every hospital door, hoping, praying, loving, and surviving. This is our story. And I give it to you with integrity, vulnerability, and an open heart.

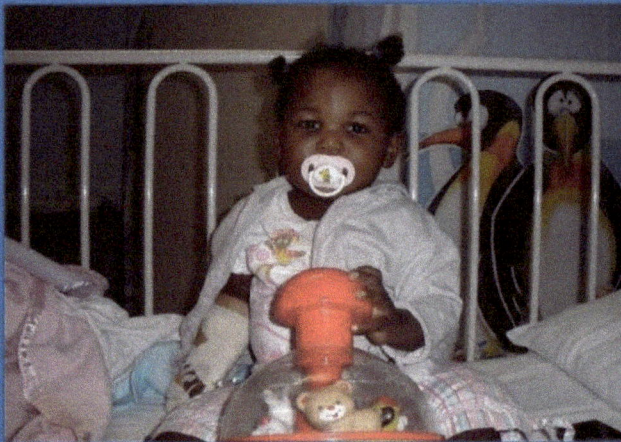

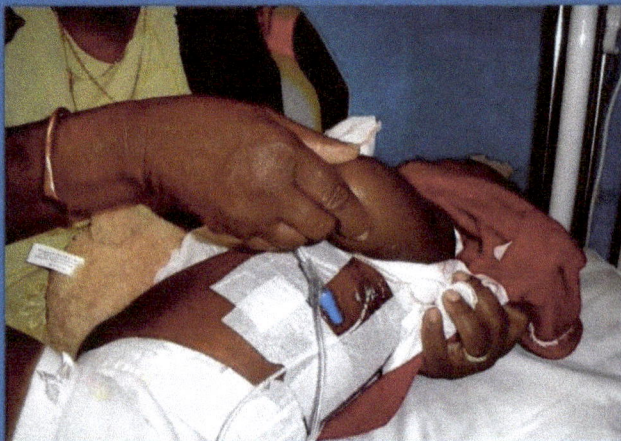

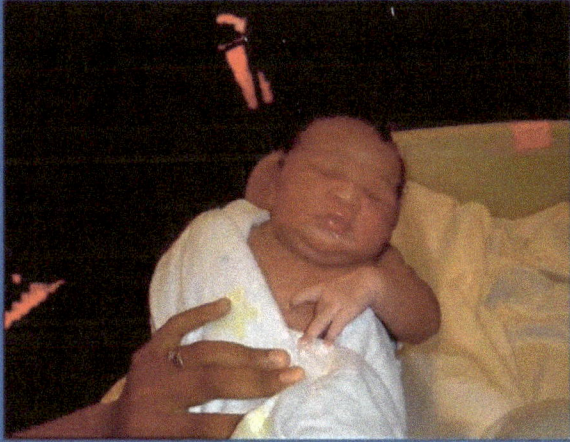

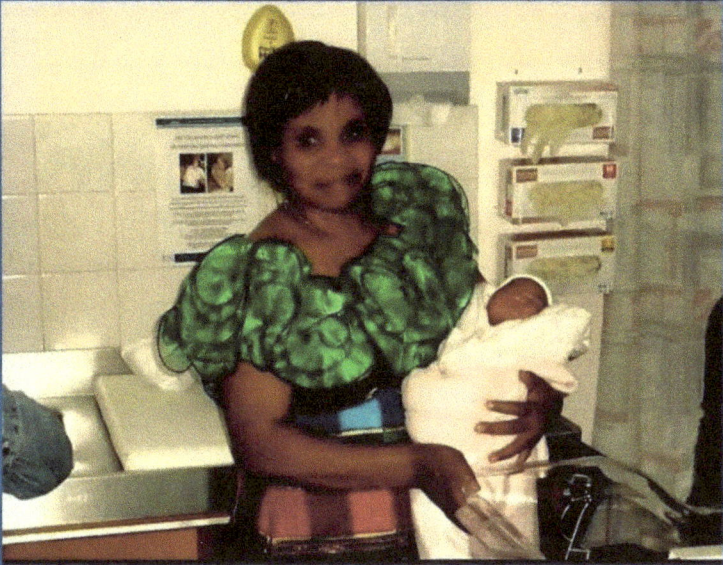

1

When the Mum Becomes the Patient

When our daughter was diagnosed with sickle cell disease, I looked back to a time when I was expecting and became a victim myself of some unknown illness. When I became pregnant with my daughter, I was prepared for a certain amount of the usual discomforts: nausea, fatigue, maybe my feet swelling up big. What I never prepared for was that my pregnancy could take such a terrifying turn that I found myself fighting for life inside an intensive care unit, with doctors uncertain if I would live at all. What I also never expected was to become critically ill with complications linked to that; I was a carrier (of the sickle cell trait, not the disease). But that is precisely what happened.

I didn't know I had the sickle cell trait. It's not something I grew up with, and I never had symptoms that rang any alarm bells. It wasn't until the doctors ran blood tests while I was in the hospital that I even learned I bore that trait. The news came as a complete surprise, and doctors were unable to explain why I was unwell. Like many people, I had no idea that carrying the trait could have such, or even that pregnancy, dehydration, and low oxygen levels could turn it into the disease in extreme circumstances. Up to that point, I had lived my life in ignorance, never dreaming that something hidden in my blood would have such a profound impact on my child's life.

I was about six months pregnant when things started going wrong. To begin with, it was an insidious feeling, that of constant weariness, persistent headaches, and general weakness. I put it down to the advances in pregnancy. But the symptoms got worse. Suddenly, I had difficulty breathing, my heart raced, my chest hurt, and my temperature soared. One evening at home, I suddenly fell.

That was the start of an eight-week hospitalisation, two of which were spent in intensive care. My Haemoglobin was frighteningly low. I couldn't take a single step or speak without gasping for breath. My organs were starting to show signs of weakness, and doctors struggled to understand what was going on.

I remember being laid in a hospital bed, with a mask blurring my face. There were machines everywhere, and the sound of their distant din made me feel like I was falling further into unconsciousness. It was not long before the doctors discovered that my peculiar symptoms had been brought on by a rare complication arising out of this pregnancy, while carrying the Sickle Cell trait under stress. Any oxygen saturation levels would lead to cells in my red blood system sickling into themselves, thereby causing blockages and severe swelling throughout body tissues. This effectively resembled a crisis of sickle cell disease in which all parts of one's body have suffered damage. I found it difficult to breathe, to the point where my lungs were especially affected. They said I had acute chest syndrome, a potentially deadly condition more commonly seen in patients with sickle cell disease.

I was afraid, not just for myself but for my unborn daughter as well. Would she survive this? Could I? It was clear from the expressions on the doctors' and nurses' faces that we were in dire straits. My husband tried to remain brave, but I saw the fear in his eyes every time he visited. Family members came, prayed, and waited, each one of us grasping some shred of hope as days turned into weeks. Every hour spent in the ICU felt like an eternity. I was hooked to machines, unable to speak without them most of the time, and my body was so swollen from medications and fluid retention that I could hardly recognise myself.

But what made it worse, still, was that despite doctors having discovered while I was pregnant that I had the sickle cell trait, no one ever sat us down to explain what that might mean for our baby. There were no serious discussions, no referrals, no mention of the possibility of our first child being born with a sickle cell disease, probably because my partner, too, was a carrier of the trait, something we hadn't even considered. We were never advised to come back for genetic counseling or follow-up tests. So, when, months later, we found ourselves back at the hospital, holding our sick baby, we were completely taken aback. It felt as though somebody had let us down or as if it had all been somehow predictable and might even have been avoided if only we had had proper warning. Instead, we embarked upon the most challenging period of our lives, totally unprepared.

I had moments of delirium in and out, sometimes from pain, sometimes from drugs. I still remember the nurses softly whispering, moving my body, touching that baby's heartbeat. That tiny heartbeat, regular and insistent on the monitor, became my anchor. It was the reminder of life, of hope, of persistence, and both.

After I had slowly recovered, the ICU doctors sent me back to the ward for the remaining six weeks of my hospitalisation. My body was still weak, but my soul was unyielding. I was more determined than ever to protect the new life inside me. Together, she had lived through everything with me: breathlessness, fear, pain, and uncertainty. And her strength lent me mine.

Leaving the intensive care unit after two weeks, I moved to a general maternity ward. I was left with many more questions than answers about how my body was reacting and what this could mean for our daughter. The doctors told me that I had Still's Disease. I had never heard of it before, yet there seemed to be something related to me and this disease. So, during this period of "Still's disease", I began to look further into what was happening to me. I asked questions at every visit, during every hospital stay, but the answers were always vague and incomplete. I spoke with doctors, nurses, and specialists in the hope that one of them might be able to explain why my body was reacting this way.

But what I encountered instead was uncertainty. Although I knew that I carried the trait, few medical professionals could give me an explanation for why my symptoms were so severe or any dangers that I might be facing. To date, the issue of sickle cell trait has never been raised in any tests carried out by the hospitals.

I began conducting my research by reading research articles, joining forums, and searching for people with similar experiences. Unsurprisingly, I discovered that women who have sickle cell trait carry one normal hemoglobin gene and one sickle hemoglobin gene. Most of the time, sickle cell trait does not cause illness, but pregnancy places extra demands on the body and can make some of the risks more noticeable.

Pregnant women with sickle cell trait are more likely to develop urinary tract infections, including kidney infections, compared with women who do not have the trait. Because of this, doctors often do urine cultures each trimester so that any infection can be treated early. Although sickle cell trait on its own does not usually cause severe anemia, pregnancy increases the need for iron and can lead to low blood counts, so fatigue and weakness can be more pronounced.

Sickle cell trait can also increase the chance of painless blood in the urine, and pregnancy may make this happen more often. Both pregnancy and sickle cell trait slightly increase the tendency for blood clots, especially after delivery, so your health team will often encourage you to stay hydrated and keep moving to reduce your risk. Some studies suggest that women with sickle cell trait may have a slightly higher risk of high blood pressure in pregnancy (preeclampsia), although the evidence is mixed. True sickle cell "crises" are rare in women with only the trait, but severe dehydration, low oxygen levels, or infection during pregnancy can sometimes trigger sickling events. And this is the rare position I was in, I developed all these symptoms that needed this long hospital stay.

For the baby, most studies show no large increase in miscarriage or stillbirth with sickle cell trait, although there may be a slightly higher chance of low birth weight or preterm birth. The main concern is genetic: if the baby's other parent also carries the sickle cell trait or has sickle cell disease, there is a risk the baby could inherit sickle cell disease. For this reason, genetic counselling and partner testing are recommended during pregnancy.

When I was finally discharged, although physically weak, I was mentally stronger than ever. Every breath was like a gift. My motherhood was already beginning to take shape, not just in the usual way, but on a deeply personal, medical, and emotional level. I had already paid a price and suffered so much before my daughter drew her first breath.

I have not failed to see the irony. In the last trimester of my pregnancy, I was fighting for my life only to discover that my child, too, carried both my blood type and the thing I had been immune to: sickle cell anemia. As it turned out, while my daughter was still being diagnosed, I was recovering from one crisis inspired by the trait. However, my daughter would be born with the complete condition and face its challenges. We are as close to each other as two people can get, far more than most people could understand. Both of us were fighters; we were tied together by blood, but we would have to learn to face together. I learnt from this period in my life more than any medical book could ever tell me, in that limbo where we spent one moment struggling to maintain huge blood reserves, and another feverishly trying to get some oxygen into our systems; sickle cell trait is not always benign. It was through these experiences that I learned to advocate for my health, listen to my body, and push for answers, even when they were difficult to obtain by any other means. But more than all else, my strength, hers; the strength we would have to summon as we went forth into unknown territory together.

Taking my daughter in my arms during the journey home from the hospital should have been one of the happiest moments in the world. After all that had happened to us, the complications during the pregnancy, my two weeks in intensive care, there were times when even doctors gave up hope. It just felt miraculous now to walk between those tall doors alive and with a new baby nestled at my chest.

It ought to have been pure happiness. Beneath the relief, however, was a quiet and sinking fear that went right out of those hospital doors with me: What next?

At that point, we didn't know our daughter had sickle cell disease. She looked perfect, small, drowsy, and peaceful. Her first baby checks were all good, and we were focusing on recovery, both physically and emotionally. At that time, there was no neonatal/newborn screening for sickle cell disease, nor with so much else going on, did I give it even a thought. My partner and I were both trait-carriers; yet since this was something never mentioned in our community, we were unaware of it. There were so many other worries then, and we did not get the time to read more about the effects of sickle cell trait.

We got into life domestically. I went through my trial recovering from a severe injury, after an 8-week hospital admission, delivered a baby, and pranced around trying to do everything for it. I watched over her bassinet, checking her breathing hourly, checking with Google on every sound she made, rash, and sneeze. I put that down to post-hospital admission jitters. But deep down inside, something just never quite rang right. I put it down to excessive caution.

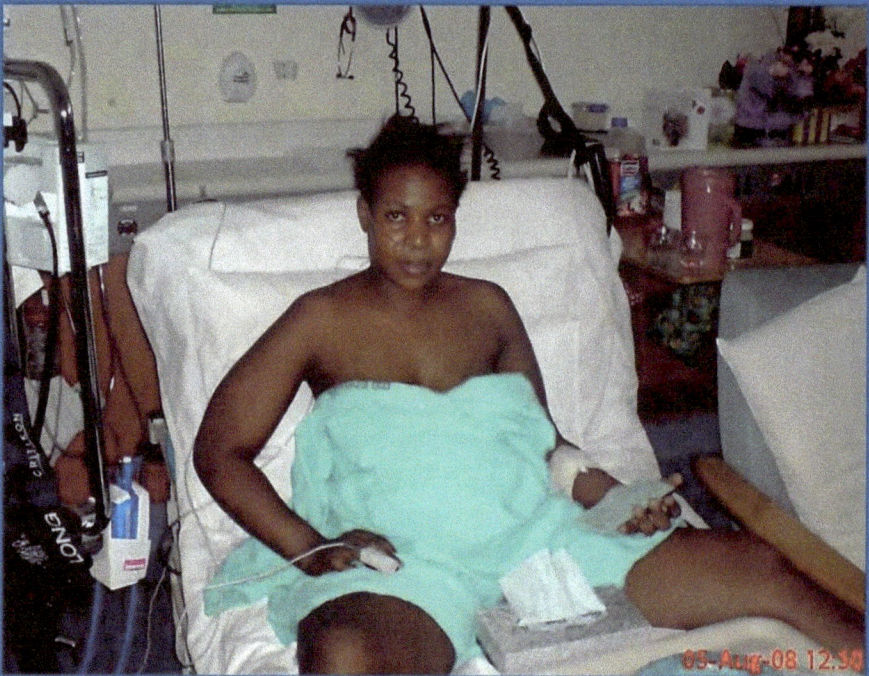

Understanding Sickle Cell Trait

When your child is diagnosed with sickle cell disease, your world shifts. Suddenly, you're facing a condition you may never have heard much about before. Doctors start talking about genetics, red blood cells, and something called "sickle cell trait." The words can feel confusing at first. You're not only trying to support your child medically and emotionally—you're also trying to understand how this happened, and what it means for your family moving forward.

Let's take a step back and gently walk through what sickle cell trait is, why it matters, and

how it fits into your family's story.

What Is Sickle Cell Trait?

Sickle cell trait is not the same as sickle cell disease. It simply means that a person carries one copy of the sickle cell gene and one normal gene for haemoglobin. This person is a carrier; they don't have the disease themselves, but they can pass the gene to their children.

To develop sickle cell disease, a child must inherit two sickle cell genes, one from each parent. If both parents have sickle cell trait, there's a 25% chance with each pregnancy that their child will have the disease, a 50% chance the child will carry the trait, and a 25% chance the child will inherit neither gene and be completely unaffected.

Most parents of children with sickle cell disease find out they carry the trait only after their child is diagnosed. This can bring a flood of emotions, confusion, guilt, and even blame. Please know you did nothing wrong. Sickle cell trait is inherited silently. You can live your entire life with the trait and never have symptoms. Many people don't even know they have it unless they are tested. This is no one's fault, it's a part of the genetic story written long before any of us could see it coming.

How Common Is Sickle Cell Trait?

Sickle cell trait is much more common than many people realize. In fact, it's estimated that:

- About 1 in 12 African Americans has the trait.
- It's also found in people of Caribbean, Indian, Middle Eastern, Mediterranean, and Latin American descent.

These numbers mean that in many communities, sickle cell trait has been quietly passed down through generations. Families may not have talked about it, or older relatives may have lived their lives unaware they carried the gene. That's why so many parents are surprised when it becomes part of their child's medical story.

Does Sickle Cell Trait Cause Health Problems?

For most people with sickle cell trait, there are no symptoms. They live normal, healthy lives and may never even think about it after finding out. However, in rare cases, especially under extreme physical conditions, the trait can cause complications. These situations might include:

- Extreme dehydration
- Very intense physical exertion, especially at high altitudes or in hot weather
- Low oxygen environments, such as during deep underwater diving or high- altitude mountain climbing

These rare complications can include pain episodes, blood in the urine, or, in very extreme and uncommon circumstances, more serious events like sudden collapse during intense exercise.

This doesn't mean that people with sickle cell trait need to avoid physical activity. Far from it, exercise is healthy and important. It just means they should be aware of their limits, stay hydrated, and avoid pushing themselves beyond endurance, particularly in hot or high-altitude environments. For children with the trait who play sports, it's wise to let coaches and teachers know, so they can watch for signs of overexertion. If you're ever in doubt, talk to your child's healthcare provider. They can give you personalized guidance and answer any specific concerns.

Why Is It Important to Know Who Has the Trait?

Knowing that you or your partner carries the sickle cell trait helps explain how your child came to have sickle cell disease. But it also has important implications for the future:

- Family Planning: If both partners carry the trait, there's a 1 in 4 chance that any future child could have the disease. Knowing this can help parents make informed choices. Some may consider genetic counseling, testing, or different family planning options.
- Informing Extended Family: If you carry the trait, it means your siblings might too. And if they're planning to have children, it could be valuable for them to get tested. This information can ripple outward to cousins, nieces, and nephews, helping others make informed decisions for their families as well.
- Understanding Your Own Health: Even if you've never had symptoms, knowing you have the trait can help you take precautions in specific situations. It's about being proactive, not fearful.

Testing for the Trait

Testing for sickle cell trait is simple and typically done with a blood test. In many countries, newborn screening includes testing for both sickle cell disease and trait. In Australia, the test is free for people on Medicare and those on certain visas. Find out from your General Practitioner if you are eligible for the free test. Very soon, Newborn screening to test for sickle cell disease will be introduced in Australia. If you're not sure whether you carry the trait, or if other family members want to find out, your doctor can help arrange testing.

It's also worth noting that having the trait does not "turn into" the disease later in life. The genetics are set at birth. You cannot develop sickle cell disease if you only carry one gene. However, understanding your carrier status is still important for your health and your family's future.

Emotions Around the Diagnosis

For many parents, finding out they have the trait only after their child's diagnosis can bring up a wave of emotions. It's normal to ask:

- "Why didn't I know sooner?"
- "Could I have prevented this?"
- "What does this mean for my other children?"

These are deeply human questions. Please hear this: You are not to blame. Genetics is not something we choose; it's something we inherit. And now that you do know, you're empowered. You have the opportunity to take steps that can protect and prepare your family. You're already doing that by seeking information and supporting your child. You are not alone. Other parents are walking this road. There are communities, doctors, and advocates who understand what you're going through and are here to help.

Moving Forward with Knowledge and Compassion

Understanding sickle cell trait is a powerful step in navigating your child's diagnosis. It adds a piece to the puzzle. It provides clarity. And it helps you become not only a caregiver, but an advocate and educator for your child, your family, and maybe even your wider community. You don't have to become a geneticist overnight. But knowing the basics, the role of the trait, how it's inherited, and how it may affect health, helps you make decisions with more confidence. The love you give your child, your presence at appointments, your commitment to learning, all of it matters deeply. You are doing something incredible in a challenging situation: you are showing up, learning, and loving fiercely. Let sickle cell trait be a chapter in your family's story, not the whole story. One that gives context, not blame. One that brings understanding, not fear. And one that helps you walk forward with strength and compassion, knowing you are doing everything in your power to give your child the best possible life.

2

The Diagnosis That Changed Everything

When you first hear the words "sickle cell disease," it can feel like a foreign language. Doctors may explain it with complicated terms, lab results, and medical charts that are overwhelming in the moment. As a parent, what you need most at the beginning is a simple, clear picture of what this illness is, how it affects your child, and what it means for your family's future.

This chapter is here to give you that picture, a personal story.

Sickle cell disease (often shortened to SCD) is a genetic blood disorder. This means it is something your child was born with, not something they caught, not something they developed later, and certainly not something caused by anything you did or didn't do during pregnancy. At its core, sickle cell disease affects the red blood cells, the part of the blood that carries oxygen all around the body.

Normally, red blood cells are round, soft, and flexible. They move easily through blood vessels, like smooth little disks sliding through a tube. In sickle cell disease, some red blood cells become shaped like a crescent moon or the blade of a sickle (that's where the name comes from). These cells are harder, stickier, and less flexible.

Because of this shape, they can:

- Clump together and block blood flow, causing what doctors call a pain crisis.
- Break apart faster than normal cells, leading to anemia (low red blood cell count).
- Cause damage to organs over time because the body isn't getting the

steady oxygen supply it needs.

Think of it this way: red blood cells are like delivery trucks carrying oxygen. In sickle cell disease, many of those trucks are damaged or stuck in traffic jams. Some deliveries never reach their destination, and over time, parts of the body suffer because of it.

Sickle cell disease is inherited, which means it's passed down through genes. Every child gets two copies of the gene that controls haemoglobin (the protein inside red blood cells that carries oxygen), one from each parent. If a child inherits one sickle cell gene and one normal gene, they have sickle cell trait. They usually don't have the disease, but they can pass the gene on. If a child inherits two sickle cell genes, one from each parent, they have sickle cell disease. Sometimes, a child may inherit one sickle gene and another type of abnormal haemoglobin gene (such as haemoglobin C or thalassemia). These variations are also considered forms of sickle cell disease, though symptoms may differ in severity.

With this in mind, here is my sickle cell disease diagnosis story!

One of the hardest parts for parents is discovering that they were both carriers and never knew. It is important to remember that being a carrier is not an illness, and no one chooses what genes they pass on. This is not your fault.

There are moments in life that divide everything into "before" and "after." For me, that moment came when I heard the words: "Your daughter has sickle cell disease." Before that, my life was filled with the excitement of becoming a mother for the fourth and last time, sleepless nights, lullabies, and dreams of my baby growing strong and healthy. After that moment, everything changed. For many families, a chronic diagnosis feels like a bomb going off, not something you see, but something you feel in every part of your being. The shockwaves ripple through your relationships, your finances, your mental health, and your sense of security. No one talks enough about this part, the way it shatters your idea of what you thought parenthood would look like. The truth is that a chronic illness doesn't just affect the child; it reshapes the entire family.

Our daughter was perfect from birth. I still remember how warm she was in my arms; her tiny hand entwined around my finger. To the outside world, she looked like any other healthy newborn. But something hidden in her blood was silently shaping her life. She was fourteen months old when her second pneumonia struck. As she was admitted to the ward, the doctor gently told us: "Your baby has sickle cell disease." My heart raced. I gripped the bed tightly, trying to prepare myself. I watched the doctor's lips move as she explained about red blood cells curling into sickles, blocking blood flow, causing pain, infections, and organ damage. I barely heard a word. The phrase "sickle cell disease" echoed endlessly in my head. I asked, "Is there a cure?" She shook her head softly. "There is no absolute cure, but with proper care, children can live full lives." I walked out of that room feeling like the ground had fallen away beneath me. That night I didn't sleep. I cried silently while holding my daughter, blaming myself, terrified of what the future would look like.

While I was in the hospital, we discovered that both my husband and I carried the sickle cell trait, something neither of us had known. We had unknowingly passed it on to her. I felt crushed with guilt. I drowned myself in medical journals, online forums, and support groups. The stories I read frightened me, but they also gave me hope, proof that children with sickle cell could grow, learn, laugh, and thrive. From then on, every detail of her life required vigilance. Every sneeze made me anxious; every fever sent us rushing to the hospital. I became not only her mother, but her advocate, caregiver, and protector. Those first months were the hardest. I had to say goodbye to the future I once imagined and build a new one. Life became structured around medicines, appointments, and precautions. Yet, in the middle of all this, there was her smile, sunlight breaking through the gloom. She reminded me daily that she was not just her illness. She was a whole person, full of curiosity, laughter, and love.

Parenting a child with a chronic illness is a 24/7 responsibility. Spontaneity disappears. Every outing, school day, or holiday must be carefully planned. This constant vigilance is exhausting, a quiet form of trauma. Families often drift apart under the strain. Communication breaks down. Couples cope differently; one dives into research, the other withdraws. Sometimes blame creeps in, as if genetics were anyone's fault. The extended family may not understand, leaving you feeling isolated even in a house full of people. The financial strain is real. Hospital visits, medications, time off work, and travel costs pile up. Many caregivers are forced to cut back or quit work. The anxiety of never feeling secure financially weighs heavily. Siblings feel the impact too. They notice the hospital visits, the missed birthdays, the exhaustion on your face. Some hide their feelings to avoid burdening you; others act out. They, too, are navigating grief and confusion. And through it all, parents often neglect their own mental health. Depression, anxiety, and burnout are common, but many of us feel we can't afford to break down. Yet caring for ourselves is not a luxury; it's essential. You cannot pour from an empty cup.

Despite the fear and exhaustion, I also discovered resilience I never knew I had. I became her champion, her voice when the medical system didn't listen, her advocate when her pain wasn't taken seriously. We faced ignorance, even from some doctors who dismissed her symptoms or downplayed the seriousness of sickle cell. I learned to fight for her care, to demand that her fevers and pain were treated urgently. Slowly, I began to trust my instincts again. And in the middle of appointments and crises, there were moments of grace. Her laugh, her first day at school, her play with friends, each moment became sacred. Her joy taught me to live in the present, to find gratitude even when the future felt uncertain. Through support groups, I found other parents walking this road. Their stories reminded me that while sickle cell is invisible to many, we are not alone. In their strength, I found my own.

Sickle cell disease changed our family forever, but shattered doesn't mean destroyed. Over time, we began to rebuild differently, but not less beautifully. We found new strength, new allies, new purpose. My daughter showed me daily that she is not her diagnosis. She is brave, resilient, and full of life. She dances in the kitchen, hugs her grandparents, and holds onto her favourite toys as treasures. She is living proof that joy and illness can exist side by side. I no longer see myself only as a mother; I see myself as an advocate, a learner, and a fighter. Sickle cell has forced me to grow in ways I never expected. It has taught me that love is stronger than fear, that hope can survive the hardest nights, and that family is not defined by what we lose, but by how we keep showing up for one another.

A diagnosis like this changes everything, but it doesn't have to break everything. What comes after the shattering is not about going back; it's about becoming who you need to be, together. Because love doesn't quit, and neither will we.

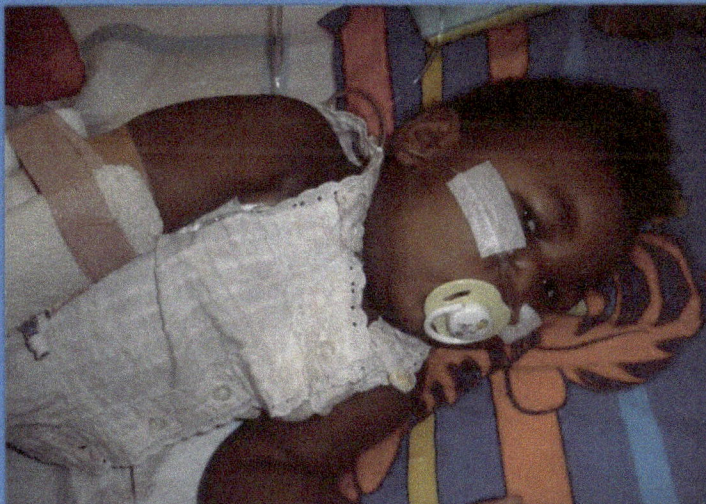

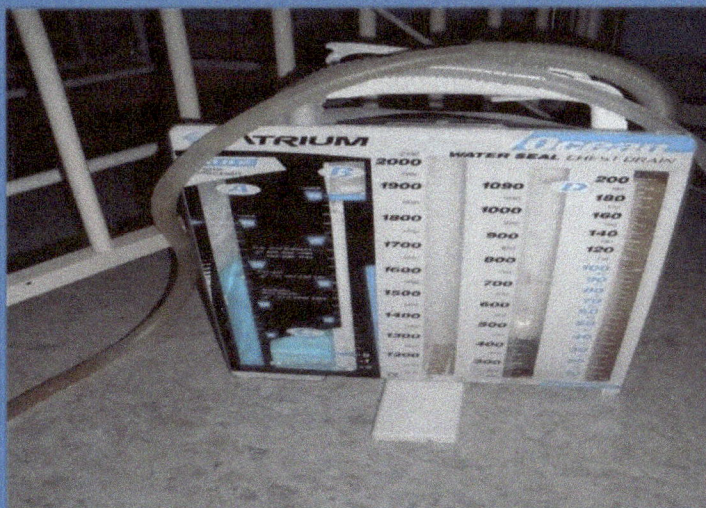

3

When Sickle Cell Shows Its Face

Nothing prepared me for the first pain crisis post the acute chest syndrome that made us know she has sickle cell disease.

By that time, I had read about them, listened to other mothers speak, and watched videos on what to expect. But reading and reality are never the same. When it happened, when my daughter began to cry in that high-pitched, unfamiliar way, I knew something was wrong, but I didn't realize how bad. Until then, she had been relatively well, growing steadily, hitting her milestones, charming everyone with her giggles. But that day was different. She had been cranky since morning. Her appetite dropped. She didn't want to be held, but she didn't want to be put down either. When I touched her legs gently while changing her nappy, she screamed a cry I had never heard from her before. My heart dropped.

I took her temperature: 37.8°C. Not quite a fever, but my instincts were shouting at me. I gave her fluids, rocked her, and tried to soothe her, but her cries became louder, more desperate. That night, her temperature spiked to 38.5°C, and her hands and feet felt cold and swollen. I rushed her to the emergency department, heart pounding with every red light I stopped at.

At the hospital, doctors confirmed what I feared: she was experiencing her first vaso- occlusive pain crisis. Her red blood cells were sickling and clogging her blood vessels, cutting off oxygen and blood flow to her limbs. The pain, even in an infant, was excruciating. She was given pain relief and fluids, and we were admitted for monitoring.

That was the first of many.

Over time, I learned how to spot the subtle signs before a crisis took complete control: a change in her mood, a sudden lack of energy, unusual crying, or swelling in her hands or feet. I also began developing my list of home-based remedies and strategies, not as replacements for medical care, but as a mother's first line of defence.

My Regular Treatments and Home Observations:

1. Hydration Is Key

I religiously had her drink. What helped, too, was that she was always thirsty, hence hydration for her was very easy. Thirst can lead to crisis; therefore, I made sure to always have a cup or syringe available for her to drink water, diluted natural juice, or breast milk. When she didn't feel like drinking, I'd feed her small sips of fluids with a cup or syringe. In hot weather, we doubled our liquid intake and avoided the heat at noon.

2. Warm Baths and Compresses

When she began to suffer the initial pain or stiffness, I gave her a warm bath. I wouldn't make the water too hot, just enough so it could relax her muscles. Gentle plays in the water massaged away constraints. Following the bath, any areas or spots that she pointed to indicate trouble were wrapped in a warm towel, then a compress was added.

3. Soft Movement and Stretching

When her legs or arms seemed stiff, I gave some soothing words and gentle movements to help blood flow. I played games with her or recited songs, getting her to kick and stretch her limbs as she lay on her back. But I never forced anything on her, we just followed wherever she led me.

4. Rest, But Not Too Much

I allowed her to sleep when necessary but advocated for some light activity once the pain had subsided. I found that being too still for too long sometimes tended to worsen circulation, so I alternated rest with gentle movement, such as hugging, soft rubbing, or light stretching.

5.   Tracking Symptoms in Writing

I developed a simple symptom diary, which includes the date, what she did, temperature, liquid intake, and signs of any new pain. Patterns emerged, enabling me to predict her symptoms more accurately as well as explain them better when we ran aground in an emergency room.

6.   Slowing Down the Inflammation

With her doctor's agreement, I explored natural means to balance her weakened immune response and decrease inflammation. I made warm ginger tea (at about four times the necessary dilution), employed bone broths, and pureed everything for their content. Of course, everything was checked with her team.

7.   Establishing a Peaceful Atmosphere

This can be especially true for children: stress can be a significant trigger for crises. I designed a quiet, soothing, and predictable room for her. I used lullabies, sensory toys that emitted lovely scents, and a small hug before bedtime (with lots of hugs throughout the day). I chose to give her away when the weddings were over, not exchange gifts.

However well I looked after her at home, there came moments when we had to take a trip to the hospital. And every emergency visit had its little bit of human pain, hastily packing up, flying through traffic, answering the same questions repeatedly, yet trying to keep calm in all ways at once. We spent nights in the hospital sometimes, yet I would tuck myself into a chair beside her crib, one hand always on her.

The most painful part was watching her try to understand why she was in such agony. As she grew older, her questions grew more intense: *Mummy, why does my body hurt? Why do I have to go to the hospital again? How long must I endure this?* The truth was that I sometimes didn't have answers.

I also experienced difficult moments at the hospital whenn staff were unable to comprehend just how much pain she was in or when we had to wait too long for medication. I had to fight bitterly at times to make myself heard, even raising my voice on occasion and demanding escalation. I learned never to minimise anything observed at home. No one knows her better than I do.

I had backup care in place for her, just in case I had to work through the night, but neither of those scenarios happened. It was a continual exercise in dualism, of keeping life normal while being ready at a moment's notice for something unexpected. But in the medical chaos, I would cling to every good moment. Every month that she went pain-free would mean a private little party in my heart. Every week free of hospital visits brought delight like cherries on an untold amount of cake. A whole night without getting up for emergencies was an object of rejoicing, which I wanted to make into an esquire and a duke who never lifted his cap.

When a crisis came and went, I'd think to myself that it was just one more tempest in our lives. Not everyone had such luck. The key factor at that time was community. When I found other mums, we could share ideas. It was suitable for both one's feelings and practical advice. I learned what some parents did and told my account in turn. I began to help new parents with the diagnosis, sharing my home management techniques and hospital packing lists as well as offering tips on what to say to children about their condition.

Finally, my daughter remained most assuredly strong throughout. She learned to put her pain into words that were hers. She knew when to say, "Mummy, my leg hurts" or "I feel tight in my body." She was getting her voice, a little go-getter who had faced more than most children her age yet still smiled cheerfully every day. Was that at all difficult for us? The pain crises and belly were a harsh reminder of the havoc sickle cell disease could wreak. But they also showed the power, instinct, and indomitability that lay inside us both.

4

Finding Our New Normal

There is a period of calm after every storm. This is the first time you look up and see that the clouds have moved on, albeit only for a short while. We eventually found a way to rhythm in our lives, not letting sickle cell disease overshadow every aspect of living. Although it wasn't perfect, that understanding became our new standard.

By the time my daughter was around two years old, we had been through more than most families experience in a lifetime. Several hospital admissions. Numerous crises of pain. Late nights when she couldn't sleep. But along with all those hardships came growth. I no longer trembled at the mention of her diagnosis; I had grown to understand her cues and mannerisms, shifts in her mood. When she needed me to drink more, what things might keep her home from daycare, and when to pack that hospital bag just in case.

But each year added new layers to life. She was gradually becoming her little person, curious, talkative, joyful. And with her growing independence came new challenges for us both: getting her into a day nursery and helping her find friends her own age.

The Initiation Into School With Sickle Cell Disease

I agonised over the decision to enroll her in preschool. I worried about germs, physical play, temperature control in classrooms, and how well teachers would understand her condition. Would they notice if she were getting dehydrated? Would they dismiss her if she said she was in pain? Would she be left out of activities that were too strenuous?

Before her first day, I requested a meeting with the school. I came prepared with her medical plan, emergency contacts, a folder of printouts about sickle cell disease, and a detailed list of her signs and symptoms. I explained what a pain crisis might look like, what to do in an emergency, and the importance of regular hydration and breaks from physical exertion. I also made sure her teachers knew the difference between a child who's just tired and one whose body is signalling a deeper problem.

To my surprise, the school was receptive. They assigned her a "care buddy," a teacher who would do daily check-ins. We worked together to create a care plan. They always allowed her to carry a water bottle and gave her rest breaks when she needed them. I even supplied a small "comfort box" for the classroom: a soft blanket, colouring books, and a pair of warm socks for cold days.

Despite all my worries, she thrived. She loved learning. She made friends. And most importantly, she began to gain confidence in expressing her feelings. Watching her grow into a child who could say, "I need a break" or "My body feels tired" was a victory I didn't take for granted.

Healing Homes

Living with a chronically sick child changes your home from a place of mere eating, drinking, and sleeping to the site of a battlefield, a retreat, and your first, sometimes only, way to treat. The longer I had to manage our home so that it supported her health, both physically and mentally, as well as spiritually, the more I understood its influence on her quality of life. Today, many of these practices remind us how to stay calm, escaping crisis mode.

Here are some home cures and wellness practices that helped to maintain both balance and frequency of crises effectively.

Hydration Station

We incorporated water into her daily routine. I set up a hydration station in the kitchen, complete with comical cups, a bright water dispenser, and star stickers for each cup she drank. Occasionally, I would add lemon or cucumber to give the water a taste, as we know sickle cell warriors may be fussy eaters at times. During the colder months, juice was replaced with warm fluids (caffeine-free and doctor-approved). Dehydration is a leading cause of crisis, so even the days she didn't feel like it had to be taken seriously.

Herbal Baths

When she was aching or tired, I would occasionally give her a hot bath steeped with Epsom salts, lavender, and a few drops of eucalyptus oil. When she took these baths, it was about more than just relaxing her muscles or easing the pain in her bones. It was also a rare moment of peace, storytelling, and communication. She came through at ease and satisfied, feeling that the tension of life had been loosened, and as light as possible.

Massage and The Gentle Touch

I began to add a gentle massage to my daughter´s daily bedtime routine, focusing on her legs, arms, and back: warm olive or coconut oil infused with the scent of a little diluted clove or ginger oil. I used cold and massage to help her poor circulation. This let me check for any swelling or tightness that might not have been noticed in time. It became our moment of peace, a time when she could feel safe and taken care.

Food As Medicine

We concentrated on meals to build up her immune system, energy, and help her produce red blood cells. Spinach, lentils, and beetroot became staples in our home. I made smoothies with bananas, dates, oats, and even her favourite fruits, all things that provide strength and nutrition in their natural form. I added turmeric, a natural anti-inflammatory, into soups and curries. Every recipe was carefully planned, but always made to feel joyful and comforting.

Aromatherapy and Care

I filled the air with tranquil aromas: lavender for sleep, and citrus to instill optimism in patients who felt sterile and lifeless all around. She learnt the basics of breath training to help her state of mind when anxiety surfaced, or else she couldn't get enough air into her lungs. Every night before bed, we practised three deep breaths together. "Smell the flower, blow out the candle," I'd say. At first, she giggled, but over time, this became an emotional support for her.

Warm, Always

Her joints would feel the cold keenly, so I often wrapped her up even more snugly. Whenever we travelled by car, there were always extra blankets in the boot, spare socks, and a small hot water bottle. I made rice bags from old cloth, which were sewn into heat pads that could be microwaved repeatedly, bringing comfort.

Rest As a Healing Practice

Rest wasn't just for when she was sick; it was part of our prevention plan. I stopped comparing her energy levels to other kids. Some days she needed more sleep, more quiet time. I learned to say no to too many activities. "Slowing down is also growing," I'd remind myself.

The Emotional Burden of Chronic Disease

While tending to her body was like a full-time job, maintaining her mental health was just as important. Chronic illnesses eat away at a child's self-esteem. Watching others run faster and experience fewer days missed from school was like stabs in her heart, even if she did not say it all the time.

We've been discussing her condition with her since she was young. I never want her to feel either ashamed or perplexed. I told her in a straightforward, affectionate manner: "Your blood's just a little bit different in shape. Sometimes this makes your body work harder." I never said the words "broken" or "weak." I always told her, "Your body is strong, and we are learning together how to take care of it."

Art became another way to communicate. We drew what her blood looked like under a microscope, wrote poems together, and even acted out little stories with the red blood cells as superheroes who were fighting their way through tight tunnels. "My blood goes on adventures with Mommy," she once said. That way of thinking helped transform her body from a mere burden to something integral to the full richness of her life's story.

Joy in the Ordinary

Despite the weight of her condition, I was determined that she should have a happy childhood. We left room for laughter, music, dance, and nonsense. I let her make a mess in the kitchen. We built forts in the living room and danced around the parlour in our nightwear.

I also cut myself some slack. I realised I couldn't pour from an empty cup. I began to accept people's offers of help by allowing them to assist me, and I said yes when friends asked if they could cook for me. A feeling of guilt when I was in even greater need than usual was something that I set aside. Being the mother of a chronically ill child doesn't mean being superhuman, let alone invulnerable. It means being fully present, resilient, and honest.

The New Normal, Reimagined

Initially, our lives seemed all right. There was a framework in place, a social network, and confidence in dealing with the health care system. Sickle cell was there, clear as day, but it no longer dominated our every minute pleasure freely. It became something we lived with, not under. Naturally smooth. Of course, challenges remained. We had unexpected flare-ups. She sometimes couldn't go to school on account of it, and hospitals were still visited. But now, they didn't shake us quite as deeply. We had tools, faith, and most importantly, we had each other. Finding our new normal didn't mean an end to pain, but it did mean a beginning of peace. A peace not founded upon certainty but rather upon being prepared, loved, and strong together. And it was in this peace that my girl thrived, not despite sickle cell, but because of it. The new normal, redefined.

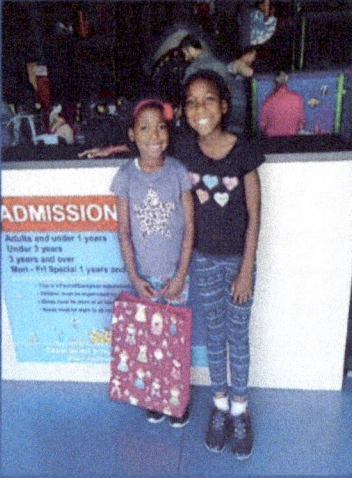

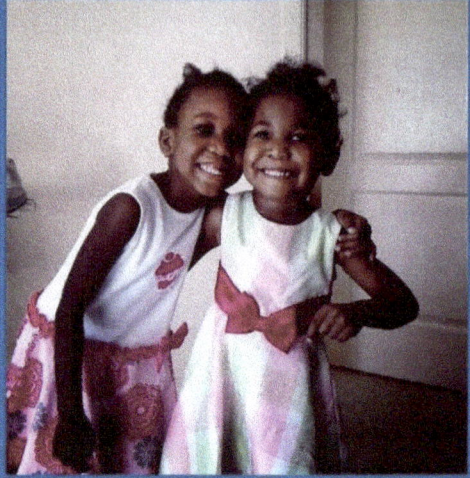

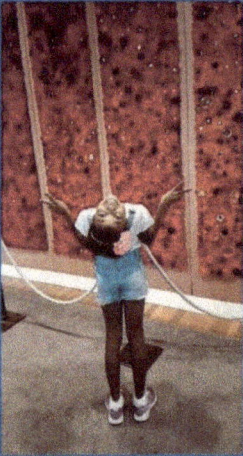

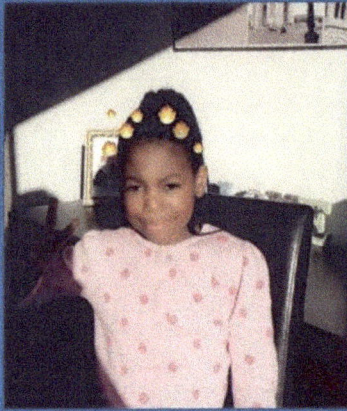

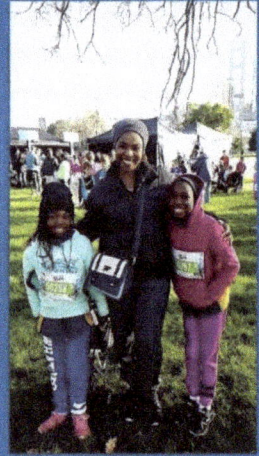

5

Life With Sickle Cell Disease

Living with sickle cell disease is a complex, ever-changing journey. It influences every moment of daily life, not only for the diagnosed child but also for the entire family. As a mother who has walked this path with her daughter, I've learned that managing sickle cell involves as much vigilance and planning as it does love, resilience, and flexibility.

The unpredictability of sickle cell disease can be overwhelming. One day, your child could be energetic and romping around, but the next, they might crawl into bed crying and shaking with pain! For these things, your child needs both medical treatment appropriate to their condition and great patience as well as practical support services.

In this chapter, I'll share with you the practical tips and lessons learned from real families that helped us navigate day-to-day challenges and construct a life where sickle cell disease was part, but not all, of our story.

1. The Power of Routine: Creating a Back drop of Messy Life

One of the first and most important lessons I learned was the value of routine. For children with sickle cell disease, routine is not just about order; it's an essential line of defense against complications. Sickle cell crises are often caused by factors such as dehydration, fatigue, stress, and sudden temperature changes. By adhering to daily habits, this set of potential triggers is reduced for the human body, leading to greater resistance.

2. Essentials of Our Daily Lives

- A good sleep: With the help of this rule, we hope my daughter will get at least 8 to 9 hours of sleep. To make it easier for her to go to sleep at night, we started establishing a regular bedtime routine and reading aloud from her favourite book. The lights dimmed, and soft Hawaiian music played in the background, helping to relax our tired brains. We tried to avoid watching TV before bedtime, as TV screens emit too much blue light, which can be disruptive early on when everyone is learning self-discipline.

- Hydration: Maintaining fluids helps the blood to thin, and sickle cells are less likely to form. My daughter takes a water bottle everywhere, even up to today. We set alarms to remind us to drink water at regular intervals throughout the day, particularly while we are in school. I also suggested she sip water gradually, rather than guzzling it all at once. Her school periodically reminded her to drink water.

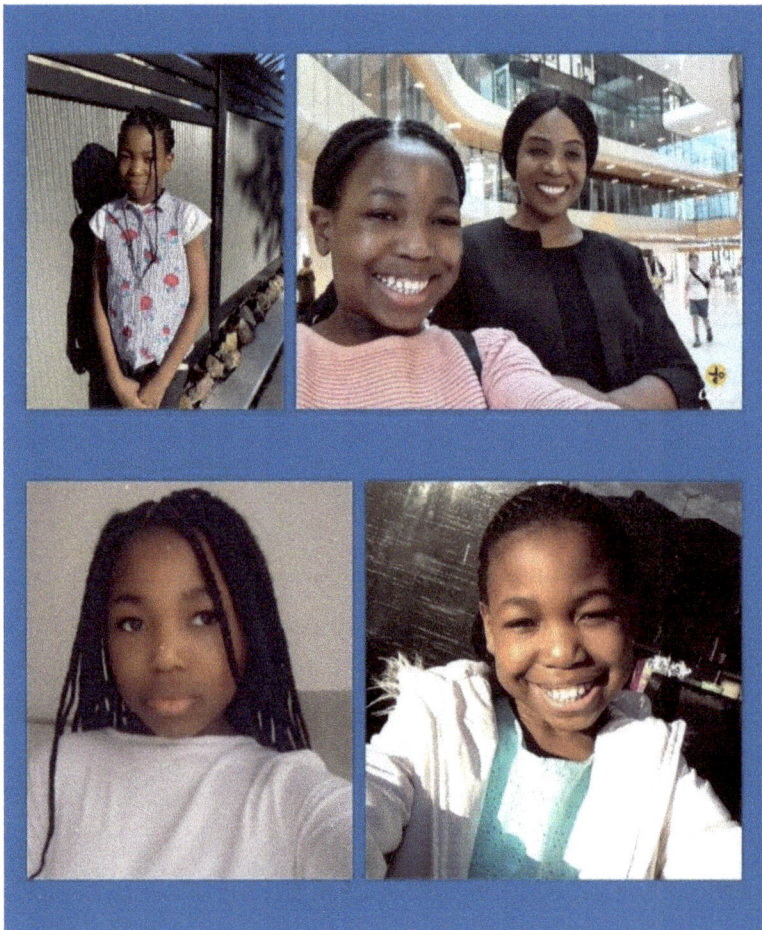

- Good nutrition is essential for healthy blood cells. We put dark leafy greens, including spinach and kale, beans, nuts, and fruits into her meals. For a quicker nutrition boost, breakfast smoothies were made from fruits and greens. I made her favourite soups from scratch, comforting, warming, and gentle on her tummy on moderate sick days. At some stage, she did have an iron overload from frequent transfusions. So, we minimised high-iron meat that she was served once in a while. Fizzy / sugary drinks gave her stomach crises, so we never had fizzy drinks in our house for over a decade. You need to know what your child's triggers are and eliminate the crises. That was how we discovered that fizzy drinks brought about a stomach crisis, which resulted in a visit to the emergency department every time she drank a fizzy drink.

- Exercise: Exercise must be done regularly, but a crisis may occur if overdone. We promoted light activity, such as swimming and walking, but balanced it with plenty of rest. I grew to understand her energy and respect her boundaries. We didn't take her out in the cold without appropriate dressing, because cold is a trigger for her.

- Flexibility Within Routine: Even in routine, it's essential to remain flexible. She would often need additional sleep or, some days, develop an inconsistent appetite. I learned to be very attentive to her body and respond to her needs sensitively and appropriately. The balance between structure and adaptability was essential.

3. Developing a Sixth Sense: Spotting Early Signs of a Crisis

Over time, I developed what many parents call a "mother's instinct," a deep sensitivity to subtle changes that often precede a pain crisis or complication.

Signs to Watch For:
- New mood swings or irritability
- Mild aches and pain, particularly in the joints or stomach
- Fatigue or difficulty concentrating
- Lack of interest in food or excessive drinking

- Cold, clammy skin or shivering
- Minor puffiness in the hands or feet
- Difficulty breathing or shortness of breath or rapid breathing

These faint signs were warning symptoms that a crisis might be brewing. Early detection of these determined infections enabled us to act quickly.

Early Interventions

- Give warm packs or heat pads to lessen pain.
- Promote early rehydration with water or oral rehydration solutions.
- Give a calm and serene place to sleep.
- Etc: for taking medication against the pain as recommended by her doctor
- Keep a symptom diary and monitor for changes to show your doctor.

4.   At Home With Pain: The Soothing and Companionship of the 'Greatest Cane'

For many people living with sickle cell disease, pain is always a reminder of their disease. Effectively maintaining it at home can avoid hospitalisation by increasing the quality of Life.

Medication Management

We pursued the haematologist's recommended treatment regimen. Paracetamol or ibuprofen could relieve mild pain. The more potent painkillers were only used in the prescribed amount. We posted a list of the meds we gave her regularly, along with an updated dosing schedule, on the fridge.

Non-Pharmacological Comfort Measures

- Heat: Baths and heating pads on sore joints were a treasure. Heat does wonders in opening up blood vessels and improving your circulation, which in turn helps loosen up muscles.
- Massage: Sensitive massage was effective in soothing muscle spasms and providing emotional comfort.
- Distraction: Sometimes the best medicine was a favourite book, music,

or a movie. Distracting her mind with other activities gave her something to concentrate on besides the pain.

- Posture: No hunching or leaning, and a comfortable sitting or lying position helped to minimize swelling and discomfort.

When to Seek Emergency Care

We always had clear guidance from our medical team on when home management was no longer sufficient and we needed hospital care. Elevated pain, shortness of breath, and neurological symptoms justified immediate assessment.

5. Get Ready for the Unexpected: Emergency Plans and Hospitals

Despite judicious management, some crises necessitate inpatient care. Planning ahead of time helped reduce the stress of these emergencies.

Our Emergency Kit Includes:

- A replica of her medical records, including the latest lab results and treatment regimens
- List of all current medications and allergies
- Contact numbers for our haematologist, GP, and hospital in case of emergency
- Warm blankets and comfortable clothing
- Favourite comforting objects like a teddy bear or a book
- Portable phone charger and snacks

Having those things packed and ready always gave me peace of mind. We distributed information on triggers and desired treatment methods previously formulated by the haematologist to the hospital staff.

Building Resilience

We built resilience with positive affirmations, mindfulness exercises, and celebrating little wins. Resilience doesn't mean you have to go on as if pain doesn't matter, but rather, you learn how to live with pain and remain deeply engaged in your own life.

6.   Tech to Keep You Organised and Informed

The introduction of technology in modern medicine has become a valuable tool in our daily routines. We used apps to manage chronic illnesses, prompting us to log our symptoms, medication times, and hydration. I found this information useful during medical appointments. Virtual visits saved time and reduced the risk of infection during stable periods. Participating in online support groups connected us with families worldwide, where we could seek advice and emotional support.

7.   Home and Cultural Cures: Augmenting the Healing Process by Stephen Barrett, M.D.

Modern medicine is essential, but home remedies rooted in cultural practices offer comfort and a sense of empowerment.

Some Remedies We Found Helpful:

- Minerva: Anti-inflammatory ginger tea Minerva offered relief from mild discomfort and queasiness. We made new ginger with lemon and honey all the time.
- Turmeric: This spice contains natural anti-inflammatory compounds, so it was included in the diet to enhance flavour and provide medicinal benefits.
- Hot baths with Epsom salts help relax muscles and reduce stress.
- Honey and Lemon: A honey-and-lemon mixture is soothing for sore throats and supportive of the immune system.

Safety First, we always discussed home remedies with our doctor to avoid potential interactions with any prescribed medications.

8.   Transitioning Independence

As children grow, their needs evolve. We need to prepare them for those transitions, from starting school to the crossover into adolescence and eventually adulthood. I introduced my daughter to the knowledge of her condition at a young age. Teaching her how to recognise symptoms, communicate her needs, and take charge of her medications gave her confidence and independence. The shift to adult healthcare services was carefully planned over the years. We supported her treatment and care alongside her doctors. One of the biggest challenges lies in making the transition from pediatric to adult healthcare.

A Few Pointers to Smooth Transition

- Start Early: Talk and plan about transferring many years in advance.
- Educate Your Child: They should learn to understand their condition and talk with healthcare providers openly.
- Coordinate Both Teams and Their Functions: Make sure that people from the pediatric team and those on the adult team communicate to have continuity of care.
- Encourage Independence: Gradually help children take increasing responsibility for setting up appointments and managing medications.

9.   Finding Joy and Celebrating Life

We experienced hardships on the way, but there was happiness too.

We celebrated birthdays, health days, and hospital discharge anniversaries with special traditions. These celebrations provided us with strength and hope. Through hobbies like art, music, or reading, my daughter found happiness beyond her illness. Family rituals, shared meals, and togetherness served as anchors during difficult times. Caring for individuals with sickle cell disease daily is a complex dance that requires vigilance, flexibility, medical care, cultural wisdom, protection, and empowerment.

There were days of agony and doubt, and days of comedy and glory. Each of the steps, battles, and victories contributed to our story. For the families who tread this path, know that you are not alone. With love, preparation, and knowledge, a life can be crafted where sickle cell disease is part of the journey, not the destination.

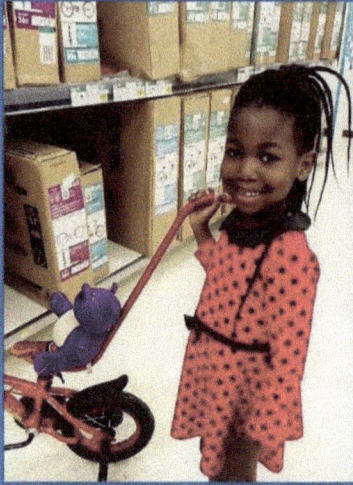

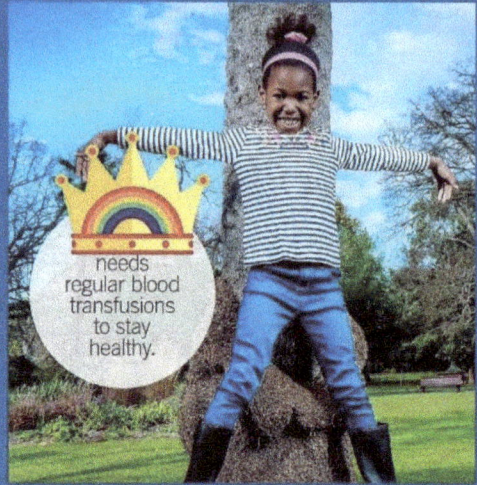

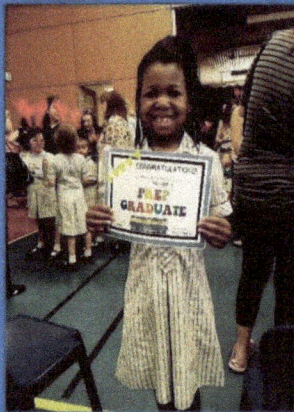

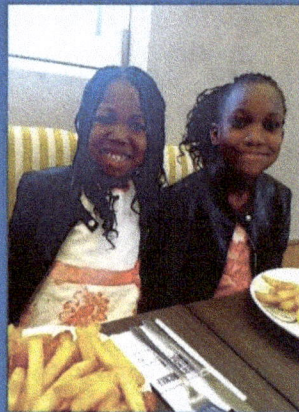

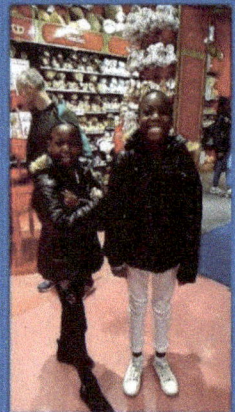

6

Navigating the Healthcare System

When my daughter was diagnosed with sickle cell, entering the world of hospitals, specialists, treatments, and medical terminology was confusing and overwhelming. I quickly realised that to provide the best care for my children, I had to do more than be a mother; I also needed to be an informed advocate, navigator, and sometimes a strong negotiator within the healthcare system.

Navigating the health system for a child with a chronic condition like sickle cell disease feels like walking into a maze. It requires multiple providers, frequent appointments, emergency visits, complex treatments, and often incongruent advice. I slowly discovered methods to make this journey less scary and more empowering for both of us.

In this chapter, I provide tips on approaching the healthcare system, working with

medical teams, and advocating for your child's needs.

1.   Understanding the Healthcare Landscape

Care for individuals with sickle cell disease is frequently multifaceted, involving haematology, general practice, pain management, nursing, social work, psychology, and, at times, surgery or transplant. Coordinated care between these professionals is essential.

Key Providers You'll Encounter:

- Haematologist: A physician who specialises in blood disorders, including overseeing treatment for sickle cell and medications such as hydroxyurea and managing transfusions
- General Practitioner: Monitors health, gives vaccines, and refers to other

services

- Pain Management Team: Attends to chronic and acute pain episodes
- Psychologist / Counsellor: Assists with emotional and mental health
- Social Worker: Helps with access to resources, financial aid, and support services
- Emergency Department: Provide acute crisis care in the hospital system.
- Post-transplant physicians, if a bone marrow transplant looks feasible

2. Building Your Medical Team: Communication Is Key

Your most important asset can be a strong, communicative relationship between you and your medical team.

Suggestions for Building Effective Relationships:

- Prepare for Meetings: Keep a health diary to note symptoms, pain episodes, medicines, and any questions you have. Bring this to appointments to convey information with clarity.
- Ask Questions: Ask for further explanation without fear. The language of medical science is not always easily understood on one hearing or reading. "Can you put that in simpler terms?" is a good question.
- Report: Your observations are beneficial as a carer parent. Record any changes in patient condition, however small they may seem.
- Request that your provider write out care instructions. Having documented treatment plans and protocols in place ensures everyone involved in care is informed.
- Keep contact details readily accessible. Store your haematologist's direct contact information. GP and emergency contacts should be in a secure location where they can be easily reached.

3. Coordinating Multiple Appointments

For children with sickle cell disease, seeing multiple doctors in one day may be overwhelming.

Strategies to Manage Appointments:

- Whenever possible, arrange appointments on the same day to reduce travel time and minimize missed school hours.
- Use a calendar or day planner. Record any forthcoming appointments,

checks, and medication refills.

- Prepare Your Child: Inform your child about what is in store so that they are not anxious.
- Look for Support Services: Some hospitals employ patient navigators or case managers who can help coordinate care.

4.   Advocating for Your Child

You are the strongest supporter of your child. You may need to query decisions or seek a second opinion.

- Know Your Rights: Understand the healthcare policies and your child's entitlements.
- Be Assertive but Polite: Clear communication helps establish partnerships rather than conflicts.
- Involve a support circle: Coming with a family member or friend will bring encouragement and can help the facts not slip your mind.
- Ask for Cultural Competence: If staff do not comprehend your culture, ask for language interpreters or services appropriate to your culture.

5.   Managing Emergency Care

Pain episodes can arrive suddenly. Emergency care must function effectively.

- Create a Crisis Plan: Work with your medical team to plan out clearly when emergency treatment is needed, what to expect, and what treatment will be given.
- Tell Local Hospitals: If you live far from a major centre where patients are looked after regularly in the event of emergencies, make sure that contact is made with your local ED in time for the details on your child's condition to be posted out in advance.
- Carry Medical Information: Having a card or record in your wallet noting sickle cell disease will speed up emergency care.
- Be prepared for bbattles: With sickle cell disease, acute pain is often underestimated in the rigors of a medical emergency. Keep calm, but insistent in asking for sufficient measures to take care of the pain.

6.   Understanding Treatments and Options

Navigating the complex web of potential treatments can be overwhelming.

Some Common Treatments Are:

- Blood Transfusions and Red Cell Exchange: The primary uses of this treatment are for severe anemia. Mostly, blood transfusions are given to maintain an acceptable haematocrit level, and this prevents complications such as strokes.
- Bone Marrow Transplant: This is a possible cure for sickle cell, but it carries significant risks, and getting ready for it is difficult (for example, long-term transplant engraftment).
- Gene Therapy: Gene therapy is a new, promising treatment for sickle cell disease. It works by altering or correcting the faulty gene that causes the disease, allowing the body to produce healthy red blood cells. This means fewer painful crises, fewer hospital visits, and a better quality of life. Gene therapy for sickle cell disease was first used in patients around 2017, and in 2023, the first gene therapy treatments (like Casgevy and Lyfgenia) were officially approved for use in the U.S. and U.K. While it's still a relatively new treatment and not yet suitable for everyone, it offers hope for a long-term cure in some individuals. Always talk to your child's doctor to understand if gene therapy might be right for them.

Before starting any of these treatments or multiple therapies not covered elsewhere in this guide, discuss the risks, benefits, and monitoring requirements of each treatment thoroughly with your medical team.

7.   Useful Personnel Information to Know in the Healthcare System

With help from Support Services and Resources, healthcare navigation encompasses not only doctors and hospitals but also social support.

Some Useful Personnel Are:

- Social Workers: These professionals can connect patients to financial aid, counselling services, respite care, and housing assistance.
- Patient Advocacy Groups: These organizations offer information, community, and they work to influence policy.
- Mental Health Services: People with chronic illness are at higher risk for mental health problems, so professional help should be sought whenever necessary.
- Educational Support: Work with your local school system to develop learning plans and provide accommodations.

8. Use Easy-to-Understand Medical Language and Documents

Medical language can be a puzzle to read.

Uncover the Medical Lingo:

- Providers may be asked to put things in simple terms.
- Mingle with the reliable online resources that your healthcare team says are up to snuff.
- Keep all test results, various letters, and your treatment plans well-organised, and provide handy copies to refer to as needed. The healthcare system can be exhausting for caregivers.

Self-care Strategies:

- Join support groups for caregivers.
- Use respite care services when available.
- Get regular check-ups for your health.
- Try relaxation and stress-reduction techniques like meditation and exercise or follow hobbies that involve natural hand movements.

When my daughter was first diagnosed, I felt overwhelmed and did not know what to expect from hospital routines and medical terms. I often found myself at appointments questioning whether my concerns were heard. Eventually, I was taking organized notes and preparing questions in advance. I also began asking for written care plans.

Once, during a hospital visit, my daughter was in terrible pain. So great was her suffering that the staff overlooked it entirely. I stood up to them firmly and demanded that she be given the proper medication, reminding them about her history. That moment taught me the importance of speaking up for her needs.

As relationships with her haematologist and care team became more trusting over time, our experience expanded. Her patience and understanding grew, too; I became more confident in dealing with care issues and treatment options as well as responding intelligently to emergencies.

Navigating the healthcare system is a critical part of taking care of a child with sickle cell disease. Although it may seem daunting and complex, acquiring knowledge, building relationships, and fighting for your child's rights will guarantee they receive top-notch care.

Don't forget, you're not alone. Healthcare providers want to work with you as their partner on this journey. With determination and courage, we can together navigate the system to ensure your child's health and welfare.

7
Emotional Journeys and Rollercoasters

Living with sickle cell disease involves managing physical symptoms, painful crises, hospital stays, medications, and treatments. But beneath these obvious challenges lies a complex emotional journey that affects anyone living with sickle cell and their entire family. Because of the chronic nature of sickle cell disease, the unpredictability of crises, and the uncertainty about treatment outcomes, the experience is filled with hope, fear, grief, and unwavering resilience.

As a mother who has travelled down this path take it seriously to say a few words. For us, the true emotions of fear, hope, and the countless struggles that lie ahead were as much a part of her condition; we had to learn how to deal with them and how mental health is inseparable from the physical aspect of having sickle cell disease.

1.   The Emotional Landscape: Fear, Hope, and Uncertainty

When my daughter was first diagnosed, my emotions were a whirlwind of shock, fear, pain, and hope. I was caught between wanting to shield her from pain, yet knowing that this was not possible. Each hospital visit served as both a grim reminder of the severity of her illness and a new opportunity for hope—hope that effective treatments would emerge, hope for days without pain and, eventually, an end to the disease.

The uncertainty was incredible. What would her life be like? Could she go to school? How could she bear such pain? These questions tortured me and shaped my thoughts and decisions every day.

Yet during fear, hope sprang up. For every significant point, whether it was a week without pain, a successful treatment, or even a happy moment, there was a beacon. Hope nourished us in the few long nights spent in hospital corridors and times when we were desperate and alone.

2. The Emotional Impact on Children

The physical condition brings an emotional load, and children with sickle-cell disease must confront two kinds of difficulties. For many, the unseen burden of chronic illness includes feeling isolated, frustrated, and anxious.

My daughter often felt different. Sometimes, when friends ran and played, she needed to sit out or avoid getting cold and tired. Missing school during crises was painful; besides worrying about being academically behind, she also feared being overlooked socially. Her anxiety was further exacerbated by fear of pain and hospital procedures. Needlesticks, blood tests, and occasional hospital admissions could be frightening; she didn't understand what was going on. It was crucial to create a space where she could safely express her feelings. We talked with her about the fears and frustrations she had harboured during these long years, and sometimes simply knowing someone hears your feelings can make all the difference. Support for siblings and extended family is vital.

3. Chronic illness affects everyone in the family.

Siblings often experience a confusing mix of jealousy, guilt, anger, and sometimes neglect as attention shifts to the sick child. My daughter's older brother would occasionally misbehave or become sullen. But once I understood that he needed just as much attention, kindness, and knowledge as I did, he became cooperative again. So, we tried to include him in our conversations, celebrate his achievements, and spend quality time with him.

Extended family members were also impacted. Some didn't know how to help or understand the disease. Guiding family members and friends became a necessary part of our journey, helping us build a stronger support network for the future, with an emotional impact on parents and caregivers.

4. The emotional burden on parents and caregivers can be deep.

I suffered from waves of guilt, feeling frustrated or overwhelmed, and wondering if I was really doing enough. Anxiety about the next crisis always affected my partner: I was also physically and mentally tired all along.

Ways of Coping to Assist Me: Seeking Support

Through involvement in support groups, I met others who were treading similar paths. Sharing experiences and receiving encouragement relieved feelings of isolation.

Professional Counseling

Therapy helped me to deal with grief, anxiety, and a sense of helplessness. It gave concrete methods for coping with stress.

Self-Care

I realised that taking care of my physical and mental health was not an indulgence, but necessary. Regular exercise, hobbies, and having friends helped fill my gas tank.

- Calm and Meditation: In particular, deep breathing, meditation, and yoga all proved useful for alleviating moments of acute stress.
- Spiritual Practice: Faith brought me comfort, hope, and strength during difficult times.

5. Recognising and Treating Mental Health Issues

Children with chronic illness are more likely to suffer from mental health problems, such as depression or anxiety. These conditions can intensify pain perception, hinder treatment adherence, and affect overall quality of life.

Signs to Look For

- Prolonged sadness or irritability

- Anti-social withdrawal

- Changes in appetite or sleep
- Lapse of attention
- Loss of interest in school or social activities

- Physical symptoms (e.g., headaches, stomach-aches) with no apparent cause

- Expressions of hopelessness for future life or thoughts about self-harm

Early intervention is essential. Trained mental health professionals familiar with pediatric chronic illness can offer support tailored to the child's specific needs.

Mental health care should be integrated with sickle cell disease care in the community, and the community must engage altogether in this systemic issue.

With the close collaboration of our doctor, my daughter's care plan now includes counseling and psychological support. The approach helps attend to both the physical and emotional aspects of disease.

6. Integrating Mental Health Care Into Sickle Cell Management

What Worked for Us

- Regular Counseling: Psychotherapy provided tools for anxiety management and coping with pain.
- Family Therapy: Supporting the whole family helped improve communication and collective coping strategies.
- School Support: Engaging school counsellors ensured emotional support within the educational environment.
- Seeking Professional Support: Counsellors and psychologists with a grasp

of chronic illness were priceless. Mental health assistance was instrumental for my daughter as well as me to help manage anxiety and stress.

The mental toll of living with sickle cell is deep. Both kids and parents can feel afraid, frustrated, and isolated. Encouraging open conversations is the key. I raised my daughter to express how she feels, angry, sad, or hopeful, from a very young age, without hesitation or question. We had very frank conversations about the disease, her fears, and her dreams.

7.   The Role of Spirituality and Community Support

Faith and community offered immense strength. Our spiritual beliefs provided comfort and meaning during difficult times.

Community groups, cultural connections, and faith-based organisations also offered emotional and practical support. Being part of a community that understood our struggles helped reduce feelings of isolation.

8.   Nurturing Resilience in Children

Resilience is the ability to adapt and recover from adversity. One of my top priorities has been to help my daughter develop resilience.

We nurtured her capacity for resilience by:

- Encouraging Self-reliance: Teaching her to recognize symptoms, communicate with doctors, and manage aspects of her care gave her the tools she needed to become a whole person.
- Promoting Problem Solving: When difficult situations arose, we talked about solutions together. This gave her a sense of capability and authority.
- Celebrating Milestones: Small accomplishments, no matter how minor, raised her confidence. The same is true for the parents; at times, they were just as frightened as their children were.
- Encouraging Emotional Expression: Typing in a journal, painting, or just talking were ways to process complex feelings for her.

- Building a Supportive Environment: Family, friends, and teachers who showed understanding and encouragement made a tremendous difference.

9. Sharing Our Story: Empowerment Through Advocacy

- Initially, I hesitated to share our story publicly, fearing stigma or misunderstanding. Over time, I found that advocacy became a powerful healing tool.
- By speaking out through support groups, social media, and public forums, I connected with others, raised awareness, and gained purpose.
- Sharing our journey turned isolation into a sense of solidarity.

10. Supporting Yourself as a Caregiver

Caring for a child with sickle cell disease can feel overwhelming. Prioritising your health and wellbeing is not selfish; it's essential.

Strategies for Self-Care

- Regular medical check-ups for yourself
- Finding a support network
- Taking breaks and using respite care when possible
- Engaging in activities you enjoy
- Practicing stress management techniques

A caregiver who is healthy and supported can better care for their child.

11. Moving Forward: Compassion, Hope, and Resilience

The emotional journey is ongoing. It requires patience, self-compassion, and sometimes outside help.

What I've Learned

- Embrace all emotions without judgment.
- Reach out for support early.
- Build resilience in yourself and your child.
- Keep hope alive, it is a powerful healer.
- Connect with the community for strength.

The emotional journeys of families living with sickle cell disease are as real and vital as the physical ones. These journeys shape our strength, deepen our love, and teach us profound lessons about hope and resilience.

To parents and caregivers reading this, your feelings are valid, and your efforts are invaluable. By caring for your emotional well-being alongside your child's physical health, you build a foundation for healing and growth.

Together, we can navigate this journey with courage, compassion, and unwavering hope.

8

The Bone Marrow Transplant— Our Journey to Healing

If sickle cell disease teaches you anything, it's how to live in constant awareness, watching, sensing, and preparing. You become fluent in subtle signs: the way your child holds her arm, how long she naps, the tension in her voice, the tone of her skin. As a mother, I became her shadow, always just one breath behind her, ready to shield, to soothe, to act. But even with all the love and the best of care, the disease was relentless.

I had heard of a bone marrow transplant the first time our daughter was diagnosed in Perth, WA. At the time, the doctors decided to test all our children just to make sure none of them had sickle cell disease or had sickle cell trait. It was at that time that we were informed that, should we consider a BMT, one of our children was a 100% match.

As our daughter grew, so did the intensity and frequency of her symptoms. Pain crises became more regular. She missed school days, birthdays, and playdates. Some nights she'd wake up sobbing, legs stiff, arms curled in pain. Her resilience was inspiring, but I could see the exhaustion building in her tiny frame.

Managing the disease on a day-to-day basis was no longer enough. We needed to look ahead and find something that could offer her a future where sickle cell disease wasn't always lurking around the corner. It became clear that we had to explore more aggressive treatment options. We started the discussions with the doctors to find out if she could withstand the bone marrow transplant due to her numerous surgeries and other complications.

Hydroxyurea—the First Line of Defence

The first step was hydroxyurea, a medication often prescribed for people with moderate to severe sickle cell anemia. It works by increasing the level of fetal Haemoglobin in the bloodstream, which helps prevent sickling and thus reduces the number of crises. For me, the decision to start her on hydroxyurea was a major one. I was afraid; however, we had no choice, and I could barely understand any medical information at the time. I had to read about possible side effects after she had already been prescribed and was taking this medication.

I had a lot of questions. How would her little body take it? I also knew that her quality of life at the time had already been compromised; hence, all we had to do was trust the clinicians. The haematologist reassured us that it had been studied for decades and was considered safe and effective for children with sickle cell anemia.

We began with a low dose, and everything seemed to be fine. I was watching constantly: her mood, her appetite, and her sleep. I started to feel almost an obsession with monitoring. However, over the next few months, something began to change. The painful crises eased off; she had moved at times when previously she would have crumpled up. She was only about 24 months old, and even though she could barely express herself, she was unable to notice the changes. The non-stop crying with no apparent reason eased, and she could eat more and sleep throughout the night.

The blood counts improved, and for the first time, we were one step ahead in moving forward. Yet hydroxyurea was not a cure. It could help manage symptoms, sure, but it could not rid the illness altogether. The triggers were still there: anxiety, cold weather, dehydration, and infection. My mother's intuition had become almost a sixth sense. I could often feel something coming before she even said the words. Sometimes, this was reflected in her eyes. At other times, it was the way she asked for infusions, which was atypical for someone of her age. The tiniest limp. A flush to her cheek. Even her silence spoke volumes. When I sensed an attack was coming in, then I would act fluid, warmth, and rest are the bricks; if, however, it was needed, paracetamol, or hospital.

At the age of five, the hydroxyurea seemed to have stopped working. The increase in foetal haemoglobin, which is not affected by sickle cell disease, stopped being produced. Other complications, like being neutropenic with signs of mouth sores, were also increasing. At one point, she was having protein/blood in the urine, and even though we stopped the hydroxyurea for a few months and restarted, these side effects would not stop.

It was at that time that the haematology team introduced another option: blood transfusions. A series of regular transfusions followed. They helped to dilute the sickled cells in her bloodstream and lower the risk of complications like stroke, which is a very real threat for children suffering from this disease. Each time we would check her iron levels and blood type to see if she needed a transfusion.

Such regular transfusions, of course, left their mark on her body. We began to detect signs of early iron overload and less effective treatment. At the age of eight, the team recommended the red cell exchange transfusion technique, in which healthy donor cells replace the sickled red blood cells. This is a more efficient treatment that also inhibits iron accumulation. She also developed antibodies, making the blood selection process very difficult.

Blood exchanges were administered via IV lines on both arms and involved several hours in the hospital. It was hard and involved long days at the hospital. She was also scared. Being hooked to two IV lines in both arms, I was equally scared. But each time she came home, she seemed to be doing just that little bit better, with fewer crises and more energy. This measure of relief for her brought temporary benefits and helped to prevent strokes as well as long-term organ damage. Once more, I had to remind myself that this was not a cure. Precious time was only fleeting, but her condition remained vulnerable.

Bone Marrow Transplants: The Cure

It was the word `cure ' that came into their minds in such surroundings as hospitals.

After moving towns in search of better treatment options, the haematologist started the conversation about the curative option again, a bone marrow transplant (also known as a stem cell transplant). This would entail substituting her damaged marrow, which has been producing sickled cells all along, with healthy marrow from somebody else. When this was successful, her body would start to make normal red blood cells. That would practically rid her of the disease in every meaning of the expression.

However, it was not simple. Bone marrow transplants involve great danger, particularly in children. Graft-versus-host disease, infections, rejection, etc. For the process itself, they had to administer chemotherapy to kill off the existing marrow, spending a lot of time in isolation while new marrow grew, and many years of follow-up medical work. Most importantly, we needed a donor. Even better would be a fully matched brother (or sister), and she had her sister as a full donor, as per information given to us years earlier.

Moving Forward With Our Decision

We decided in all seriousness. As her mother, I weighed everything: her current affliction, the perils of the treatment, but also what life without sickle-cell might bring.

We met with transplant experts, nurses, and psychologists. It was a case of laying oneself bare to them: the likelihood of success, the side effects, and the what-ifs.

But what shaped my decision was more in her eyes than in the statistics. I saw how tired she was, tired of pain itself; tired of losing out, missing something. Tired of being the sick child.

One day, almost by chance, I found myself in front of the TV. A program was playing a feature about medical advances in blood disorders. A doctor was being interviewed about how she had cured a boy with aplastic anaemia using a bone marrow transplant. I sat up, heart pounding. She was articulate, compassionate, and clearly passionate about her work. Most of all, she was in Australia. Something about that moment felt important.

I quickly noted her name and began researching. After some effort, I managed to get in touch with her. She was based in another city, but she responded. I explained our daughter's diagnosis and asked if she had ever performed a bone marrow transplant for sickle cell disease. Her reply was both hopeful and sobering.

She told me that she had never performed a bone marrow transplant for sickle cell in Australia, but she had done them successfully in France, where she had trained and worked before moving here. However, to proceed with such a case here, she would need to return to France for a short refresher course, update her accreditation, and ensure the necessary support was in place back in Australia. She promised that once she returned, she would be ready to help us.

I remember feeling a strange mix of relief and apprehension. It was a lifeline, but it came with its own risks and uncertainties. A bone marrow transplant is not a small step. It's a lengthy and complex process, with significant risks including infection, graft-versus-host disease, and rejection. Yet it was the only known cure for sickle cell disease. So, we waited. And thought. And prayed.

When the haematologist returned home to Australia and told us she was ready, we did not say yes immediately. It took a couple of months to come to a decision. We wanted to be assured that fear wasn't driving us into something we'd regret. Factors in our decision were our daughter's age, her condition at the time, the potential risks, how long she'd have to be in the hospital, and the pain of loneliness.

We also thought that she might grow up free from a shadow hanging over her future like a sickle. During those months, I kept a close eye on my daughter. Her energy, her laughter, and her playfulness were unchanged. But I knew the next crisis could come at any moment. I couldn't forget the doctor's words: *It's possible. We can cure her.* And gradually, that faint possibility began to take root in my heart, growing into something more.

So, in February 2019, after a great deal of thought, prayer, and preparation, my daughter was admitted to the hospital for a bone marrow transplant.

It was long, hard work. First, she had to go through chemotherapy to prepare her body for the new marrow. It was terrible watching her go through all that, losing her hair, suffering from nausea and a loss of sense of taste. But she was brave. More courageous than we had ever given her credit for. A mix of highs and lows marked the weeks that followed the transplant. There were days when we celebrated rising blood counts and others when we watched monitors anxiously for any signs of rejection or infection. With every hurdle, however, she struggled through. Slowly, her body accepted the new cells; slowly, sickle cells disappeared from her blood.

I cried when I was finally told she didn't have sickle cell disease anymore. This little girl, who a year earlier lay gasping for breath in acute chest syndrome, felt almost unreal to me now. The disease was gone. She would no longer require daily hydroxyurea or red blood cell exchange. No more worry over every fever, no more looming threats of strokes or painful crises or hospital admission.

It takes time to recover from a transplant. There were months of isolation, follow-ups, and a careful re-entry into the real world. But she did it. We did it.

Now she is a thriving, joyful little girl, full of spirit and life. It is not her past as a patient that defines her; it's the strength, the spirit, and love that have carried her through all of these challenges. And my own life is no longer defined by fear but by a determination to give our child the best possible future.

When I look at her now, I do not just see what a so-sick little girl was once. I see a miracle. I see valour. I see grace. I know a child who pulled off the impossible because of one moment's kindness, who lucked into the right place at the right time, or who managed, through watching TV, to have a doctor speak about happy ideals. That moment changed everything.

Getting Ready for Transplant

Before transplant, preparation was arduous. Before the chemotherapy began, we needed to make sure she was as healthy as possible and protected against all hazards. Her hydroxyurea was stopped. We performed red blood cell exchanges to reduce the sickle cell load in her system. As directed by the team, she utilised natural tonics and supplements to enhance her immunity at this time.

At home, I concentrated on helping her emotionally. We read books about hospitals and healing. We discussed the operation openly in terms that she could understand. I made a countdown calendar to help her sense of time. I let her have some say in choosing pyjamas, packing her hospital bag, decorating her hospital room with family photos, and her favourite soft toys.

In my preparations, I also found worth. I searched, meditated, and shed tears. My faith and community were mentors who have gone before me and helped guide me through the process.

Finally, the moment arrived. I held her hand as she was wheeled to an early Thanksgiving transplant service. Leaning close to be heard above the din of cheers, prayers, and hymns, I mouthed, "That's right. You are brave and powerful. We are going to get through this together."

The mother's presence is crucial to the successful treatment of sickle cell anemia, whether or not other complications are added to the already heavy burden; its course can be greatly influenced by a mother's love and dedication. During those early months of her transplant, my role was to remain the unwavering mother: to keep seeing her for who she is, to have faith in myself, trust my instincts, and never forget that one day this dark journey would end in light.

I've learned the hard way that if you think treatment is just about medicine, you'll soon realise it's not. It's also about small acts: warming her socks before putting them on, adding honey to herbal tea, singing softly when blood is drawn, especially when it's not time for another painful procedure (this truly matters for her mental state), and rubbing her back when she feels spiritually down. It's about knowing when to step in and when to let help arrive on its own. All treatments are tools, but love, insight, and being present transcend tools. If she has a transplant, everything will change. But all that came before, anguish, treatments, tough mothering, was also part of the journey.

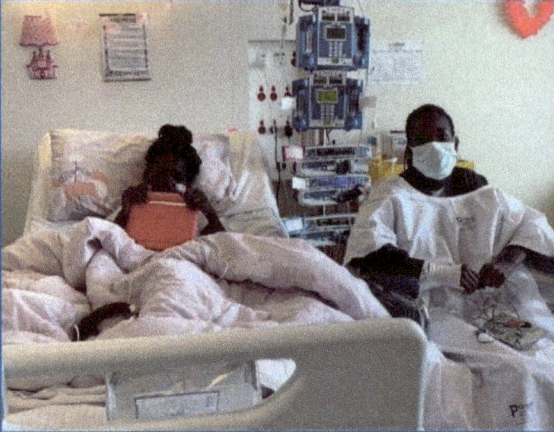
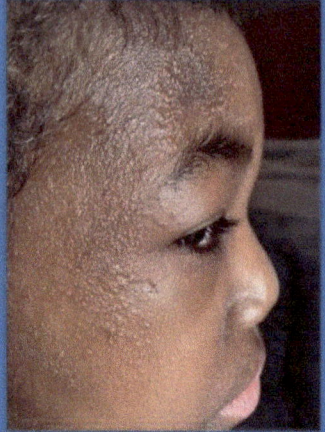
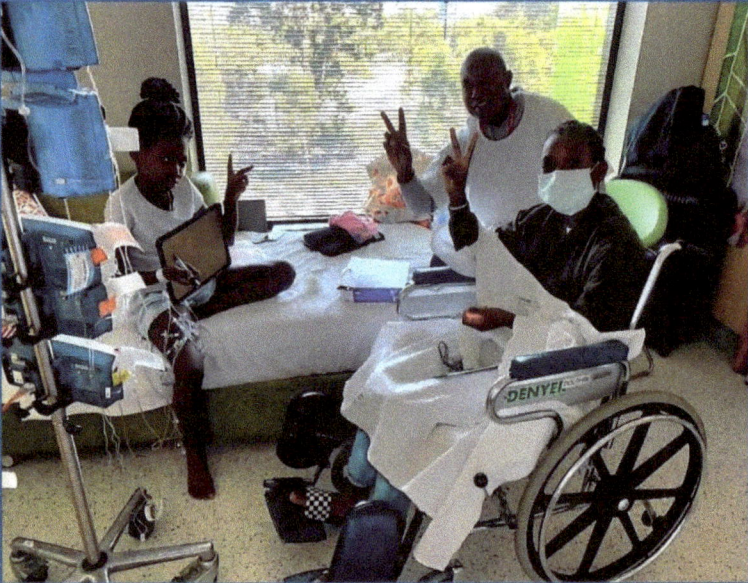

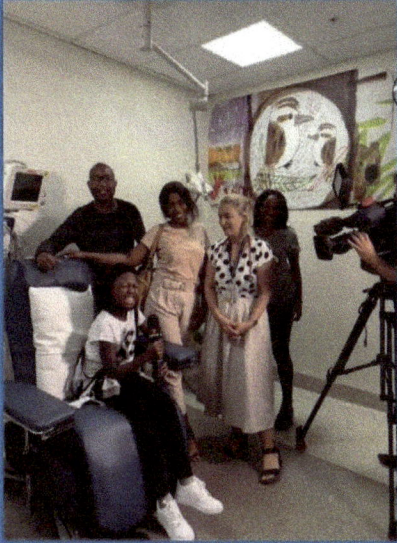

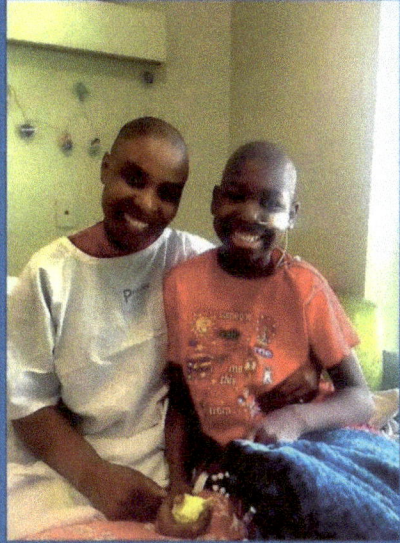

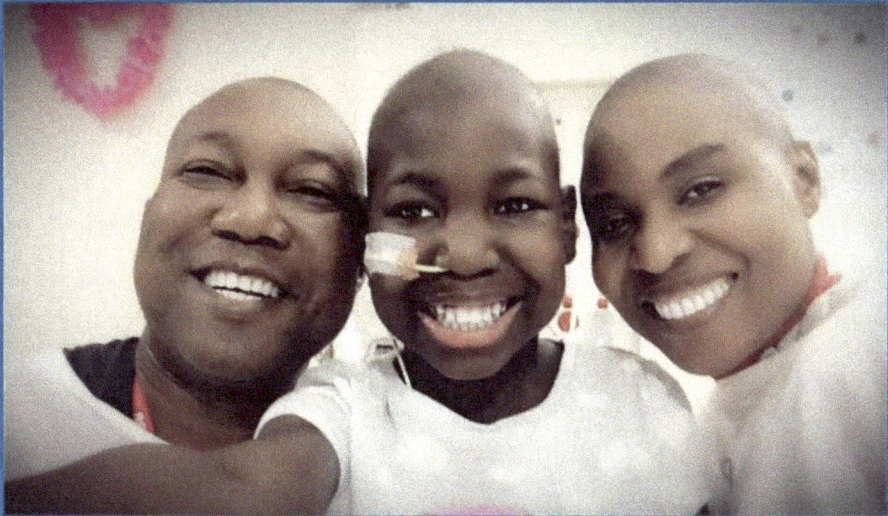

9

The Transplant, Then What?

When the day finally came for my daughter to be transplanted, it was a monumental day, an epoch in history that promised hope at long last after many years of struggling. And for every parent who has trodden this way before me, a transplant is not the end, but a whole new beginning, filled with both hardships and unexpected, rewarding experiences.

After transplantation, this chapter examines our life, including pphysical rehabilitation and emotional healing, adapting to necessities, and working toward regaining a normal childhood as well as family life.

1.   At the Beginning of Different Days, Right After Transplantation

After the transplant, the first few weeks were some of the hardest and most dangerous. With her white cell count at zero, we attended to infection control as an absolute necessity for my daughter. To shield her from germs, she was placed in a controlled environment. A sniff that was no more than just the simplest kind of cold would set off alarm bells everywhere: ''Oh no, what was that bit of phlegm? Is she running a temperature or not?'' Another scary few minutes passed for all connections.

Her energy levels were low; nausea caused by the chemotherapy and tiredness following a transplant are common side effects. Pain management was still a necessity, but it was different this time. Now the pain was often related to investigations, waiting for engraftment, and other similar procedures. This time it hurt her little body more deeply than ever before, and she had no choice but to bear it.

As a mother, I kept safety in mind. I closely monitored her daily body temperature, fluid intake, and any new symptoms. Every day brought a mix of hope and anxiety as we waited outside our children 's room to see whether there was any sign of engraftment or infection.

2.   Post Transplantation

After being released from the hospital, we would make regular visits to follow-up sessions. On these occasions, blood tests were used to assess the white cell count (the extent of engraftment). Her immune system, which had been reset, required that vaccinations be given from the ground up again. At times, the sheer number of appointments, blood yielding, and medication management became overwhelming.

3.   Handling With Care

Long-term Consequences

While a transplant was a cure for sickle cell disease, it brought along new problems.

Common long-term effects

- GVHD (Graft-versus-Host Disease): A condition is where the donor's immune cells attack recipient tissues, which can cause skin rashes, digestive problems, and even organ damage. Although we were fortunate to escape from severe GVHD, monitoring has continued over the years.
- Fertility Concerns: Chemotherapy and transplant can affect future reproductive health. Consultations with specialists helped us to understand the potential impact of all this and plan for later life.
- Growth and development: A full set of physical and mental milestones assured that my daughter was growing healthily.
- Emotional and Cognitive Effects: Concentration, memory, emotions and other aspects of life for some children experience challenges post-transplant.

## 4.	Rebuilding Immunity and Preventing Infection

One of the post-transplant's most crucial tasks was supporting immune recovery. My daughter had to dodge crowded places and keep away from sick contacts for several months. Every day, hand hygiene, clean environments, and close monitoring for any signs of infection were priorities. Her immune system required booster vaccinations slowly but steadily as it recovered. We also provided information to the school staff and her friends about her fragility.

## 5.	Returning to School and Social Life

To return to school was a major milestone for my daughter. After months of solitude with missed schooling, learning to integrate socially and succeed academically was an exercise in patience.

She faced a number of obstacles:

- working through the missed curriculum
- struggling with fatigue at school
- reconnecting with friends in the wake of an extended absence

In collaboration with schoolteachers and school counsellors, we were able to create an individualized learning program and provide psychological support.

At first, socially, she seemed shy and cautious. But with encouragement and understanding from her peers and family, she gradually found herself at home again.

## 6.	Emotional Reconciliation and Mental Health Recovery After Transplantation

The transplant procedure wasn't the conclusion of an emotional road. While the disease can be removed, both the physical and emotional scars of having sickle-cell disease remain. Both my daughter and, indeed, the whole family had to wrestle with anxiety over her health, fear of relapse, and the search for a new identity free from chronic illness.

- Continuing psychological counseling helped my daughter understand the things that had happened to her.
- Family therapy created a space where members could share feelings and rebuild relationships.
- Support groups through her peers provided links to others who had done transplants.
- Raising the level of joy and resilience is accomplished in part through such hobbies and social activities as encourage men to turn back to their "familiar" childhood pursuits.

7.   The Return of Ordinary

A "new normal" was to be established after the transplant.

This would be one entirely free from sickle cell crises but tormented with great care and vigilance over ongoing conditions. We structured our times to include taking the prescribed medication, meals, exercise, and health monitoring. The pace of family life picked up; we took to giving thanks every day, marking milestones, graduations, weddings, births, without missing a single beat, in an effort not for ourselves so much as to lift others higher. On the other hand, we knew that the transplant was a major life event, requiring careful adjustment. It was not a magical cure-all; many challenges still lie ahead.

8.   Health through body and strength building one's physical strength is a gradual process.

Muscle mass and endurance had been sapped by chemotherapy and illness; my daughter worked with physical therapists to regain her strength and mobility. We promoted regular and gentle exercise with outdoor activities as applicable.

9.   Nutrition and Holistic Care

When it comes to recovery, good nutrition plays a crucial role. We focused on foods rich in vitamins, minerals, and antioxidants to support the immune system's functions and promote repair. Hydration was still important. Holistic care, involving other therapies such as massage and relaxation techniques, helped keep stress at bay and bring about recovery:

10.   Family Relations and Roles After the Transplant

A new family relationship was formed around a transplant. The way we all went about our roles was different; my daughter became independent. She participated in and took responsibility for managing her health. Our family learnt a sense of measure between protection and freedom. We praised resilience and still recognized a need for continued care.

11.   On Looking Back: Gratitude and Growth After Transplant

With her transplant, life after transplant was a long journey, both of healing and growth. My daughter has been flourishing healthily and lively ever since. It was a long and sometimes difficult journey, but always hope-filled and beloved.

Looking to the Future: Sickle Cell and What Lies Ahead Beyond

Transplant is a question mark. For our family, it opened an inconceivable chapter. My daughter now anticipates school, friends, and activities without the cloud of illness hanging over her head all the time. We remain cautiously optimistic that life will continue to shape tests for us, but we are filled with conviction and a strong heart for facing those challenges. The second birth after a bone marrow transplant is a chance at life and health, the gift of an ocean of hope.

There are hurdles along this road, but it is a path filled with strength and healing. And at every step on that road lies discovery for yourself. As a mother, watching my daughter change has been the most moving and wonderful blessing in life. To the families out there on this same difficult path, I add my wish for wit, experience, and encouragement: You are not alone. The skies hold light at the end of the tunnel. You are not alone; the storm will pass.

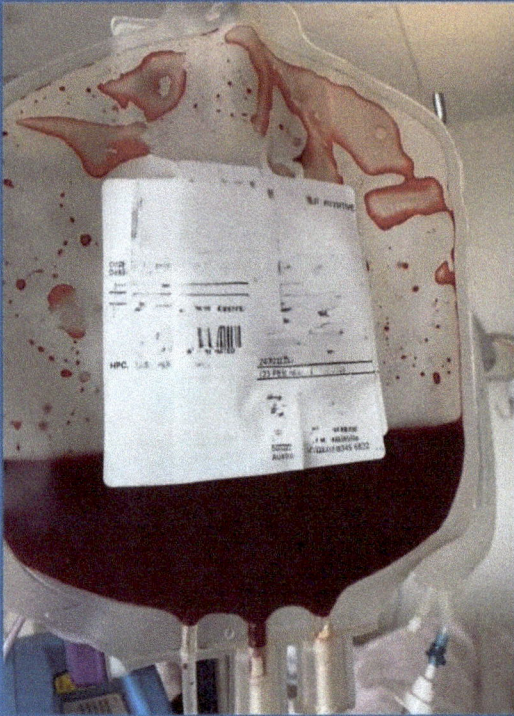
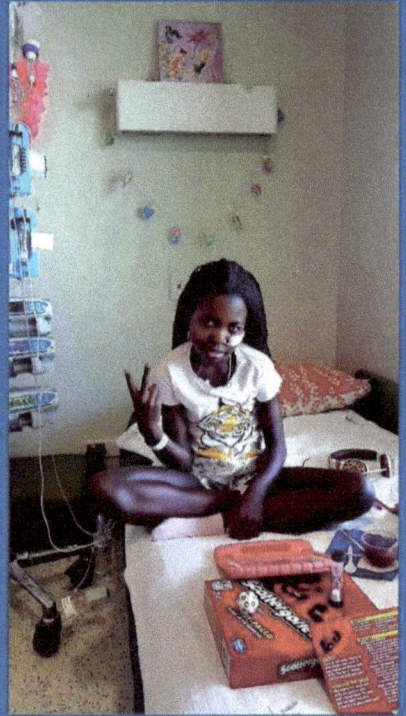

10

Becoming an Advocate—Turning Pain into Purpose

I never expected to find myself at a crossroads when my daughter was five and in care. My ten-plus years of hospital visits, sleepless nights, and public service left me emotionally and physically drained. I was pouring my heart out for her, but I felt both lucky and lonely. Living with sickle cell anemia in Australia is hard to describe. While this disease affects thousands worldwide, there are few adult warriors here to seek advice from. It seemed as if a curtain of silence had fallen over the illness, hiding its daily realities from others. I was a mother trying to navigate unfamiliar territory without a map, few guides, and only limited support.

This silence wasn't just about social withdrawal; it also made accessing necessary care, resources, and support difficult. The truth became clear early on: many people, including health professionals, had little understanding of what sickle cell disease really is. Some clinicians within the healthcare system didn't seem to understand it. I spoke with other parents about how they were being treated and misunderstood for their children. Since healthcare in Australia isn't very culturally sensitive, I found families struggling to get the care they needed. Moreover, there were no mental health resources for children and their parents, forcing them to live with this disease forever. It was a significant gap that no one seemed to address.

One of the most brutal truths I had to come to grips with was that even though my daughter suffered greatly from sickle cell disease, she was not alone. So many other children and families were in quiet struggle, fighting the same battles, but there were no places where we could gather to share ideas, help one another, or be noticed. That was when I decided that if there wasn't already a place for parents like me, one had to be created.

Lacking formal training in advocacy or technical skills, I launched a Facebook page in 2014 from our small living room. I wanted a space where parents of children with sickle cell disease in Australia could connect and support one another. I named it "Sickle Cell Support Australia." It was hard for me to get up the nerve to post much. At first, I told a handful of personal stories—the hospital stays my daughter had, those painful nights when she could not stop crying, and small victories that lifted our spirits: a good day at school or home, an easy night, a low medicinal smile.

I was surprised to see the page grow. The number of people visiting my site started to

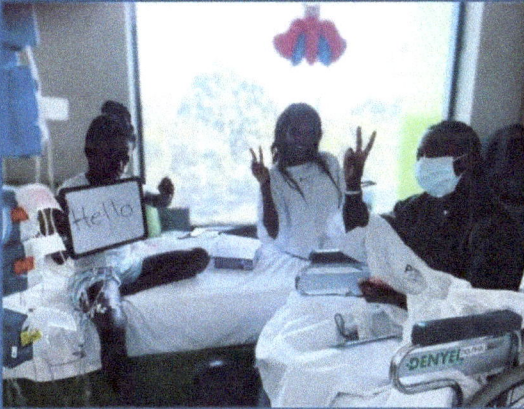
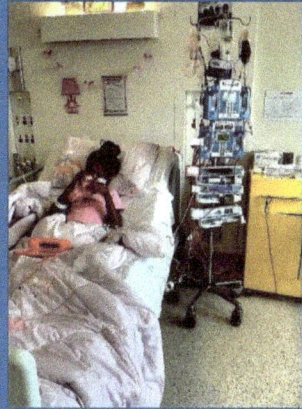
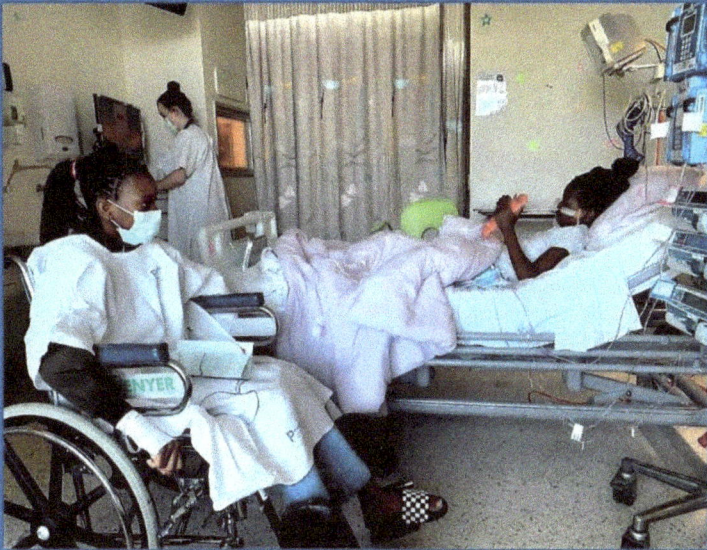

increase gradually at first, and then more quickly. Parents from all over Australia quickly joined in. They began leaving comments, sharing their stories, and asking a wide range of questions. Many had never met another family facing sickle cell disease before. For some, it was the first time they felt truly seen. The page gained a life of its own, becoming a place free from judgment, full of understanding and compassion. For me, the page was more than just a support tool. It became a lifeline. I no longer felt completely lost, and I realized that I could offer something inspiring to others who had felt as hopeless as I once did.

There is power in shared experience; only people who have gone through the same thing can truly understand you. On the Facebook page, parents found comfort and strength in knowing they were not alone. They exchanged tips about managing crises and tested these against each other's experiences, gaining new insights from monthly experts, yet they refused to let it fade away: hope born from community. Without any prior contact, mothers with children who have sickle cell disease began messaging each other. They organized local meetups and shared advice on doctors. They also started advocating for their children's rights in schools. As bonds deepened, however, our group moved beyond simple support to becoming a catalyst for change. Events like World Sickle Cell Day were now marked online together for the first time, with all our voices raised in unison. We shared vlogs, told stories, and helped others see that sickle cell disease was not just a medical term, but something that became part of our daily lives.

As the community grew, I realized there was so much more we could accomplish. Social media opened a door, but it couldn't address systemic challenges alone. I started reaching out to hospitals and healthcare providers to bridge the gap between families and medical professionals. I attended workshops, sat through conferences, and asked every question I could about how to improve care and understanding. One major challenge I often faced was the lack of resources in languages other than English. Many families affected by sickle cell disease in Australia come from African, Middle Eastern, or South Asian backgrounds. For many of them, language and cultural differences made it even harder to access or trust the medical advice they received.

To help the community better understand, we started developing culturally relevant and easy-to-understand educational materials. I believed it was important that the resources reflected my family and showed respect not just as patients but as people in front of them. I quickly realised that advocacy carried emotional baggage. As a mother, I often found it hard to balance the demands of my role as a community leader with my responsibilities. Whenever I heard a story from the hospital ward, it reminded me of something I had experienced myself.

Sometimes, mid-treatment, I wondered if I could keep going. The obstacles, such as red tape, uninvolved bureaucrats, and burnout, were very real. But every time I even thought about quitting and looked at messages from other parents, a story of hope or a small change in the hospital system would remind me why I started and why I kept going. I also learned that I didn't have to face everything alone.

Friends, family, and volunteers began offering their support. Together, we built a small but passionate team heading into 2018, committed to the idea that no family should face sickle cell disease alone. Later, after managing the Facebook page for four years and seeing the community grow, I felt it was time to turn this work into an organization with structure, resources, and greater impact. In 2018, I founded a nonprofit organisation dedicated to supporting and advocating for people with sickle cell disease in Australia.

Our aims were clear: to offer culturally sensitive training to both families and healthcare providers; to give real, as well as emotional, understanding and support to children and their parents; to turn schools, workplaces and the broader community into places where everyone is aware of sickle cell disease; and to lobby for changes in public policy which would result in not only easier access to care but also better services and continued money available for research. As we set up the organisation itself, a few challenges presented themselves. I found myself learning about governance, fundraising, grant proposals, and staying within the law. But little by little, we began to build the foundation.

With the organisation underway, we began programmes that would directly benefit families. We offered pain crisis management workshops. Teachers and school nurses received training to better understand the needs of children with sickle cell disease. We held online and in-person support groups where families could connect, share, and support one another.

We put mental health on the agenda. We realised that chronic illness doesn't only damage the body; it can lean heavily on a person's heart, soul, and mind. This led us to a partnership with counsellors familiar with the special demands of chronic pediatric disease. Healing from storytelling circles, families found a new beginning to their trauma.

Our annual events marking World Sickle Cell Day had a positive impact on the level of visibility and participation. These gatherings brought together medical experts, families, and community leaders to raise awareness about and celebrate the fight against the disease by people living with it. For many, it was the first time they had seen their experiences discussed widely in a public setting.

As we began to grow louder, we encountered public policymakers and medical institutions. We started to push for greater control over our bodies, simpler drug regimens, and more money.

For the benefit of patients with sickle cell disease in areas where we had never been present, I began sharing my family's story at conferences, in media interviews, and during consultations. Not to ask for sympathy, but to give a voice to sickle cell disease and humanize that silence.

Some things started to change. Several hospitals even arranged for coordinators to care for patients with sickle cell disease. More information became available in other languages. Awareness programs are now also mentioning sickle cell disease. However, I realize that we still have a long way to go.

Looking back, I never set out to be an advocate. It was just that I had no other choice. It was based on love and a mother's determination that her daughter, and people like her, would never again be invisible. To become an advocate has changed me in ways I'm still working out. I learned about the strength of a community, the importance of taking a culturally sensitive approach, and the power of using our voices.

I see it this way: every day, the benefits of my work go beyond helping families feel less isolated. Our organisation is still growing, reaching more people, and building new partnerships with other groups. On the healthcare side, we continue to progress with our learning programs. This is almost the same goal we set when we started a long time ago: to support families affected by sickle cell disease, break the silence around it, which often feels like a curse, and turn pain into purpose. If you're reading this as a parent feeling lost, scared, or overwhelmed, please remember, there's still hope and many positive things ahead. Together, we stay strong. Together, we can get through this.

About Australian Sickle Cell Advocacy Inc

Australian Sickle Cell Advocacy Inc (ASCA) is a national, community-driven not-for-profit organisation dedicated to improving the lives of people living with sickle cell disease and their families. Founded by advocates with personal experience of the condition, ASCA was established to respond to the pressing need for awareness, support, and advocacy for the sickle cell community in Australia.

Mission and Vision

ASCA's mission is to create a supportive environment where individuals and families affected by sickle cell disease can access the care, resources, and information they need to thrive. The organisation envisions an Australia where people living with SCD enjoy the same opportunities for health, education, and wellbeing as the wider community, free from stigma or barriers to care.

Raising Awareness

Sickle cell disease is one of the world's most common genetic conditions, yet it remains poorly understood in Australia. ASCA works tirelessly to raise public awareness about SCD, its impact, and the importance of early diagnosis and treatment. The organisation regularly engages with communities, schools, and health professionals to spread accurate information. Awareness campaigns are particularly important in multicultural communities, where many people may not know that they carry the sickle cell trait.

Advocacy and Policy Engagement

One of ASCA's core roles is to give a voice to people living with SCD in national health conversations. The organisation advocates for better access to specialist care, improved pain management, and culturally safe healthcare services. ASCA works alongside government agencies, hospitals, and research institutions to ensure that policies reflect the needs of the sickle cell community. This includes advocating for equitable access to new treatments and clinical trials, as well as supporting initiatives to increase the number of blood and bone marrow donors from diverse backgrounds. One of the most successful policy changes ASCA has advocated for is the recommendation of Newborn Screening for sickle cell disease in Australia. It took ASCA four years to successfully secure a recommendation for introducing this important screening program in Australia.

Support for Families and Patients

Living with sickle cell disease often means facing frequent hospital visits, unpredictable pain crises, and emotional strain. ASCA provides practical and emotional support to families, connecting them with resources, peer networks, and counselling services. Educational workshops, family events, and support groups give patients and caregivers a chance to share experiences and learn from each other. By building a strong community, ASCA helps families feel less isolated in their journey.

Education and Research Collaboration

ASCA recognises that education and research are key to improving outcomes for people with SCD. The organisation collaborates with universities, clinicians, and researchers to promote studies that can lead to better treatment and care models. It also provides educational resources for healthcare professionals to improve their understanding of sickle cell disease, ensuring patients receive timely and appropriate care.

Community Events and Conferences

Each year, ASCA hosts community forums and national conferences to bring together patients, caregivers, clinicians, and policymakers. These events create platforms for sharing knowledge, showcasing research, and strengthening partnerships. They also highlight the resilience of the sickle cell community and the importance of unity in driving change.

If you are affected by sickle cell disease and live in Australia, please reach out to ASCA. We are very active on social media. You can also contact me directly.

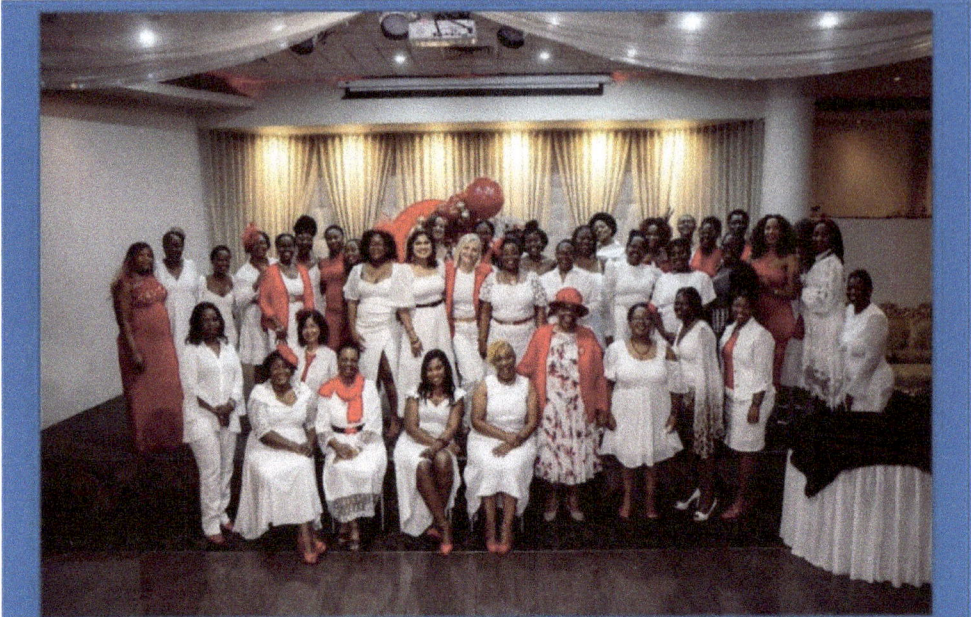

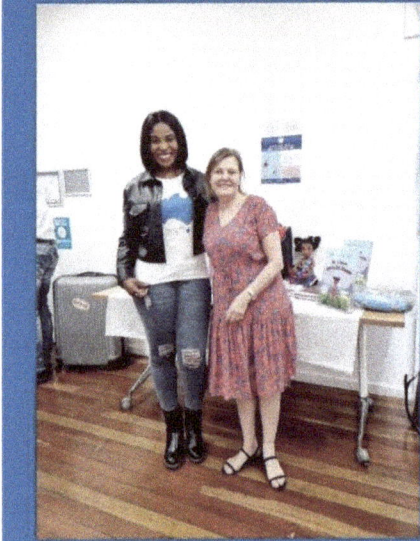

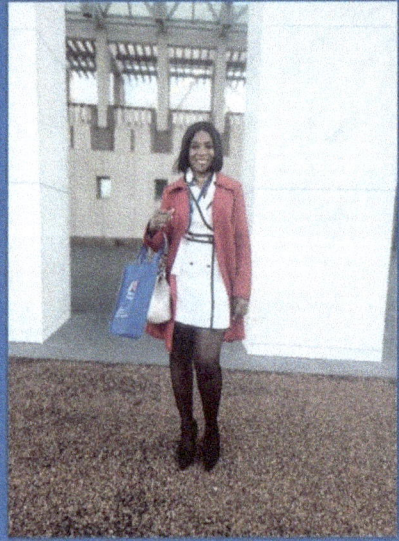

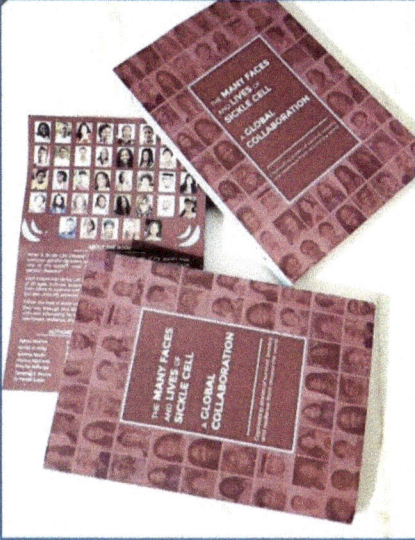

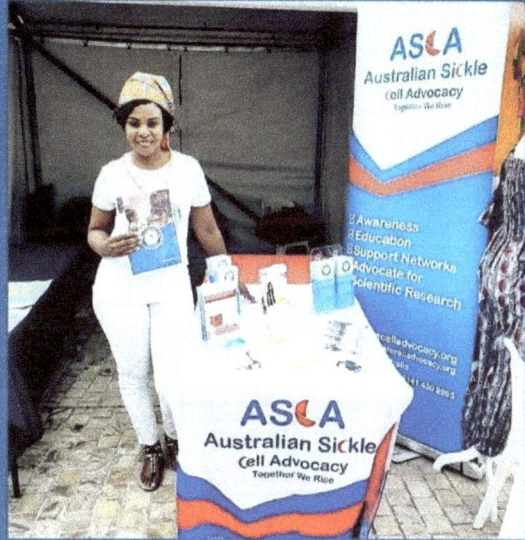

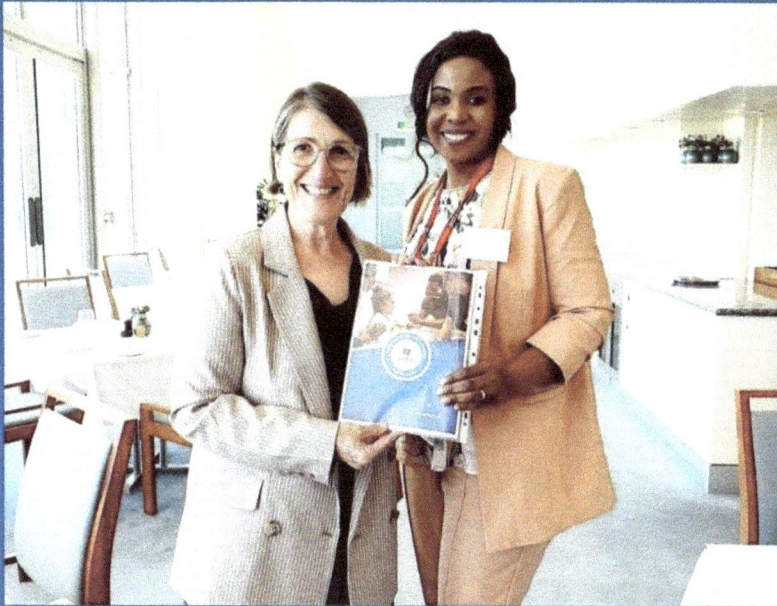

11

Raising Awareness and Community

At the beginning of my role as a caregiver for an ill child, I mainly saw sickle cell disease as a series of hospital visits and efforts to manage her symptoms. However, I quickly realised that the experience was much more complicated. Sickle cell disease affects every part of a family's life, from the physical health of family members and children's education to relationships between spouses and between parents and children. It also has a psychological impact on the entire community.

Over time, I came to see that building community and increasing awareness were not just helpful but essential. They are the foundation of our existence, and they hold the key to transforming the lives of those affected by sickle cell disease. Sickle Cell Disease is often called an "invisible illness." Unlike illnesses with visible symptoms, such as a rash, the pain and exhaustion caused by sickle cell anemia are often overlooked. Pain crises can begin or end suddenly, not indicating how one's condition can change; as a result, they are often misdiagnosed or ignored altogether.

Years later, my daughter and I experienced firsthand how a lack of awareness about sickle cell disease can affect lives. It impacted not only her medical care but also made life very difficult. Teachers mistook her fatigue for laziness. Kids avoided asking her to play because they couldn't understand her limitations.

Even within medical settings, many healthcare professionals were not always sympathetic to cultural differences and generalities; many were untrained, leading to mistreatment and criticism. Furthermore, regardless of location, some health professionals lacked proper education or appreciation of cultural variations. Sickle cell disease is often marred by prejudice and misunderstanding. It creates a major barrier: families feel lonely, unfairly treated, and ignored. That's why raising awareness is more than just sharing information; it's an act of solidarity and a challenge to create a new environment where those affected by sickle cell disease can feel comfortable.

I told anyone I could at the beginning of the movement that it took time for our family and gifts to settle in after moving. Sometimes, we spoke about our experience at schools, in community groups, or even chatting over cake at the local public pool. Once I had a 24/7 child with severe SCD, and shared the pain, hospital stays, and extraordinary emotional strain, I wanted people to see my child, not the ailment. I wanted them to realise the need for strength and survival, on what an ordinary day was like for someone who had sickle cell disease. Sometimes the back-and-forth proceeded in awkward silence, while at other times there was curiosity or sympathy. Many said they'd never heard of the disease before. That's when I realised that raising awareness isn't just something you do once and forget the conversation.

One of the most effective ways we raised awareness of sickle cell disease was through community events. Each year, on June 19, which is World Sickle Cell Day, our group sponsors a variety of activities that bring together family members, health professionals, and everyday people to participate. These events include workshops on education, cultural celebrations, and family fun days.

For example, one popular event has been the "Food Fest." At this festival, traditional meals are served representing home cultures where sickle cell disease is prevalent, to raise awareness and offer some health advice. The events are a place where children dance, grownups make connections, and physicians are available to offer guidance amidst plenty of laughter and relaxed conversation.

Through these gatherings, a space is created where sickle cell disease is no longer hidden; it is acknowledged and understood. Media coverage helps to amplify our voices, and local members of parliament have noticed. Visibility makes a difference: it helps to break stigma and brings our community some well-deserved recognition.

Providing SCD Information to Schools

Sickle cell disease is also characterised by incidents of misunderstanding or bullying toward patients by their peers. We sponsored awareness sessions where I could go and talk to the classes and the other students about sickle cell in as age-appropriate ways as possible, helping classmates build empathy and support. I also sat down with teachers, school nurses, and the principal to discuss her needs and answer questions. He continued to be proactive in keeping her safe and involved.

Schools are where children with sickle cell disease spend a lot of time, but many lack the knowledge or resources to provide proper support. We worked closely with local schools to share information about SCD with teachers and staff. This includes what sickle cell disease is, how it affects students, and what teachers can do to help. We advocated simple changes that took little time but could make a real difference; for example, being lenient with deadlines, identifying signs of fatigue, and helping set up care plans for painful episodes as the child grows. Inclusive environments in which students felt safe and supported.

After reading some of the information, a teacher said, "I didn't know anything before about this sickle cell disease, but now I see that small changes in the classroom can make a big difference." Supporting kids in school not only helps them academically but also makes them more cheerful overall and less likely to be in isolated or bullied situations.

Creating a Care Plan:

We consulted with her school to create a care plan we could put in writing, including:

- Facts about sickle cell disease and the ways it functions
- Trigger avoidance (cold, dehydration, stress)

- Warning signs educators are looking for
- Medication schedules and emergency protocols
- Contact details for emergencies

Creating Peer Support Networks

Building strong peer networks was just as crucial as raising public awareness. Our organization hosted regular support groups where families affected by sickle cell disease could connect both in person and online. In these groups, parents shared stories, offered advice, and provided support. It was a space where no one needed to explain themselves; we all understood the emotional and physical toll this disease takes. Children also formed friendships with others who saw them as individuals, not just as their illness. These connections reduced that overwhelming sense of isolation and gave many families the strength to keep going.

Harnessing Social Media's Power

Social media has become a powerful tool for connecting people, sharing information, and raising consciousness and awareness. Our Facebook page grew from a small family circle to a large, vibrant community. We use the platform to share educational content, health updates, and inspiring stories of hope and resilience. We host live online activities that invite the public to participate, combining professional advice with families seeking help. Whether their home base is five thousand miles away or just five miles, social media gives us a louder voice, amplifying our message and providing additional means for change. Of course, there are challenges with this. We had to combat misinformation, handle sensitive topics with care, and safeguard the privacy and safety of community members. We created clear guidelines that helped keep the space welcoming, allowing people to support one another in their struggles.

Collaborating With Healthcare Providers

Crucial to any improvement in outcomes was the development of partnerships with healthcare providers. We set up systems to work closely with hospitals and clinics, opening care pathways and demanding more culturally safe services. We provided training to hospital staff on the patient experience of sickle cell disease and the importance of a 360-degree approach in their treatment. We also advocated for access to hydroxyurea and bone marrow transplants, therapies that significantly transform patients' lives, as well as increased funding from society for research into sickle cell disease. By working together, we aimed to create a system that listens, thinks, and truly serves every family with sickle cell disease living in its net.

Engaging Policy-Makers

No less important was advocacy at the policy-making level. I began participating in government forums and submitting proposals that, at least tangentially, addressed better screening and financial education. Progress was slow and sometimes very frustrating. But eventually, persistence paid off. At last, sickle cell disease gained attention in both state and national health circles. Even though funding was not available for outreach programs, educational aids, and new medical initiatives, we made a concerted effort to find the necessary resources. Suddenly, the culturally and ethnically diverse communities affected by sickle cell disease were recognized and listened to.

As previously stated, one of the significant wins for our organisation was successfully advocating for the introduction of Newborn Screening for Sickle Cell Disease in the Australian Health System. After four years of lobbying for this significant development, the program was finally recommended in September 2024. As I write this, the program is in its implementation stage.

Newborn screening is a simple test performed shortly after birth to detect serious but treatable health conditions, including sickle cell disease. It helps doctors identify problems early—before symptoms appear, so babies can receive the care they need promptly.

For sickle cell disease, early diagnosis through newborn screening allows:

- Prompt medical care to prevent complications
- Early start of medications, like penicillin, to prevent infections
- Regular checkups with specialists
- Parental education on how to care for their child

Early detection can save lives and give your baby the best start to a healthy future.

What's Next for Advocacy?

As I look to the future, the focus is on building stronger systems of support, amplifying community voices, and driving lasting change in sickle cell care across Australia. One priority is expanding awareness campaigns nationwide, ensuring that more Australians understand sickle cell disease, the importance of early testing, and the value of becoming blood or bone marrow donors. Working with ASCA, we aim to strengthen its advocacy efforts, working with policymakers to secure better access to new treatments, comprehensive pain management services, and culturally safe healthcare models tailored to diverse communities. In addition, developing support programs for patients and families, such as peer mentoring, counselling, and educational workshops, will remain central to ASCA's work. Collaboration is another key step forward. By partnering with hospitals, research institutions, and international sickle cell organisations, ASCA can help bring global expertise into the Australian context. Hosting more conferences and community forums will continue to create spaces where patients, families, and professionals can share knowledge and shape future care strategies. Ultimately, ASCA's next chapter is about growth, visibility, and impact, ensuring every person living with sickle cell disease in Australia feels supported, empowered, and never left behind.

A Call to Arms

If you are a parent, patient, or friend, your voice carries weight. Get involved; tell your story. Help others and push for change. Together, we will make for a tomorrow in which nobody is alone with sickle cell. My journey from being a parent, anxious and alone, to a person with a voice and agency in the fight has been transformative. Through advocacy, suffering has become a purpose for me. Solitude became a fellowship. Hope became the spur upon which action took its starting point. I am proud of what we have achieved and eager to make efforts for the future.

Challenges On the Road

However, it hasn't been easy. There has been stigma, propaganda, and at times, apathy. Some families chose not to work with us out of fear of reprisals and a lack of trust in the healthcare system. Cultural and linguistic barriers make communication difficult, and securing funding has always been a challenge. But challenges also made us more determined. We responded by staying adaptable, listening to our community, building strong partnerships, and remaining committed to our mission.

Over the past four years, we have experienced many moments of joy and success. Parents reported improvements in their children's school performance. Young people find support and form new friendships within the network. Health workers are better educated and more compassionate.

Ultimately, policy changes have led to the creation of new resources and increased public awareness. Our greatest success is that families now feel seen, heard, and valued. We will continue advocating for more research, better cures, and ultimately, a cure itself. At the core of everything, awareness and unity mean connecting, building a community where every child with sickle cell disease is nurtured and cherished, where parents support each other, and society learns, grows, and welcomes those living with this illness. The journey of our lives has remained unbroken. I am proud to walk it alongside so many courageous families. Together, we are changing lives, breaking down barriers, opening doors, and giving true meaning to the hope that sickle cell disease will soon be something of the past.

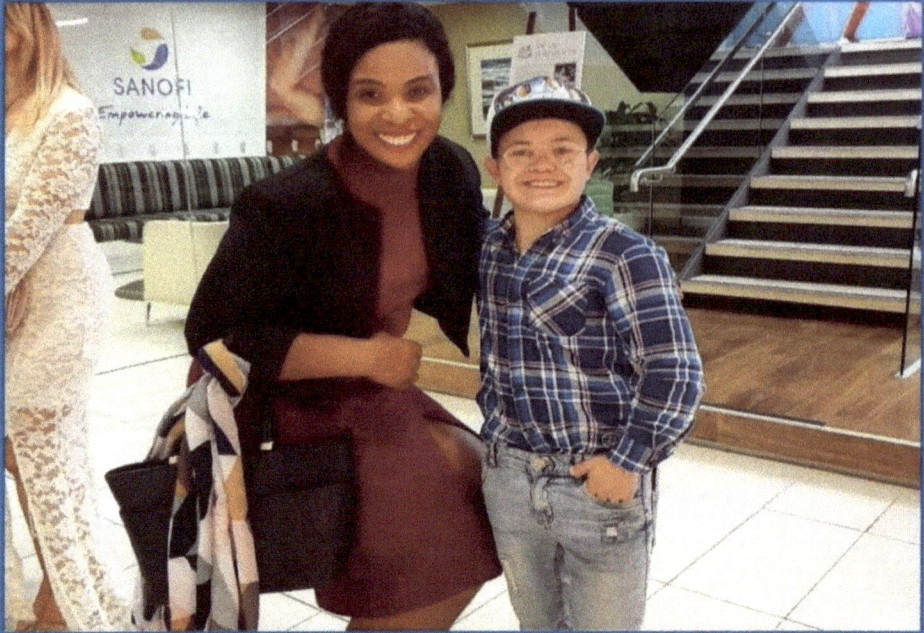

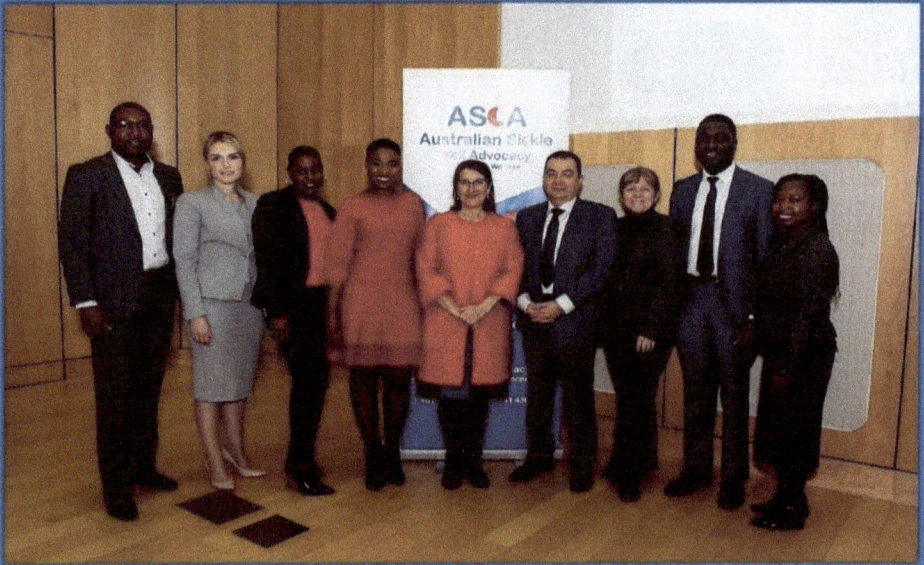

12

Advocacy, Self-Advocacy, and Awareness

Sickle cell disease has been a deeply personal journey for us, but it quickly became apparent that it was part of something much larger. Many families also partake in this story, but they keep it quiet. When my daughter was five years old, I realized we were alone. Living in Australia, a country with excellent health care, I could not find any adults living with the disease. This was a big absence. It highlights how little attention sickle cell disease receives in mainstream discussions, that so many gaps exist among community care services, or indeed cry out to be filled by those who are best equipped for this task.

In this chapter, I'll discuss how my personal experience sparked a passion for advocacy, the challenges and triumphs of building a community, and the importance of raising awareness about sickle cell disease. I hope that this chapter can inspire others to use their voices and effect change.

The concept of self-advocacy was not something I had planned to grasp; it was something that circumstances forced me to acquire. From the time that my daughter was diagnosed with sickle cell disease, I learned rapidly: Being her caregiver also meant being her voice whenever it was necessary; acting as an advocate (or even brawler) in situations where no one else even began to understand our actual situation. A few times, I was all there was between her and an institution that understood what she was going through

It was only human for me in that situation to look to the medical profession for help. I should have known that those doctors, nurses, and specialists whom we met, and surely because at first, everything seemed well with them, must have an explanation. At least my daughter's best interests would always be in their hearts, and they would continue to do what needed to be done. But I quickly discovered that while they possessed science, there could be no understanding of pain thresholds specific to her alone and other warriors, the nature and course of her crises (and that these afresh each time), even so far as it concerned whether any treatment we ever received matched up with practices elsewhere in the country or elsewhere on earth altogether. That is when I began to realise that if I did not ask questions, speak out when necessary, and never change my mind even in dire circumstances, my daughter would suffer instead!

Self-advocacy is an important part of receiving the care you need. It means, in any dialogue where your health, happiness, or future is being shaped, to ensure you protect yourself and your understanding of reality. For many people with sickle cell disease, self- advocacy is not something to be skipped; it is necessary.

Her first time in the hospital, my daughter needed to wait for a specialist to prescribe her pain medicine, even though she was clearly suffering. She lay in bed. I waited. Minutes passed. Then an hour, and still, nothing happened. I watched her curl into herself, tears soaking the pillow, her hands clenched into fists. Suddenly, something clicked inside me. I walked out of the room, found the nurse, and insisted in no uncertain terms that she get pain relief right away.

Here's what I said: The history of being prescribed drugs she had been given before; you have to act immediately with sickle cell crises brought about by pain management, and once again, try to explain to them the effects of sickle cell disease. I could see the doubt in their eyes. Nevertheless, someone listened, and they acted.

I will never forget this moment. It was not only because it brought relief to my daughter, but also because that moment opened my eyes to how important and how necessary self-advocacy is under such conditions. Lived experience is just as valuable as complex clinical data.

When she was a child, I knew my daughter better than anyone else. I could tell when a crisis was approaching, for example, just by the sound of her voice. I knew what was "normal" for her. I was able to notice the smallest changes in her looks. That instinct, combined with learned knowledge or the natural intuition of a mother, became my strongest asset.

Sometimes, self-advocacy involved directly challenging people's assumptions. For example, consider sickle cell pain. When someone arrives at an emergency room and healthcare providers unfamiliar with the disease misinterpret pain signals, question medication needs, or misclassify sick ulcers, it's likely they simply don't understand what's happening. I had to correct these misconceptions repeatedly. Sometimes, I had to print out journal articles, bring medication logs, or insist on speaking to consultants directly. Other times, I had to be persistent: to keep going despite feeling exhausted.

The hospital was not an exception. Such self-advocacy also carried through to schools, community services, and even friends and extended family. I had to explain why my daughter needed to drink water frequently and how she couldn't stay outside for very long in either cold or hot weather. I had to warn teachers that certain school activities might pose a health hazard. Teachers meant well, but they didn't always fully appreciate the seriousness of her condition. I had to educate them, not to alarm them, but to inform them. And I learned the importance of advocacy not only in a crisis, but also proactively, before problems arise.

The power of self-advocacy is in knowing. As a parent, I made it my personal responsibility to learn everything I could about sickle cell disease. I read research papers, attended medical webinars, and asked numerous questions. I kept folders of medical reports, drew up care plans, and noted down patterns in my daughter's health. I armed myself so that I could advocate effectively. The more I found out, the more confident I became in speaking up.

However, knowing what to do is not the only part of advocacy. It also involves having confidence, and this appears to be the aspect that many caregivers struggle with. We fear being labelled as a "difficult" or "pushy" parent. We worry that if we are too pushy, our children could suffer. For families from culturally and linguistically diverse (CALD) backgrounds, these fears can be intensified by language barriers, racial prejudice, or past negative experiences. In such cases, self-advocacy becomes even more essential and requires greater courage.

Perhaps the most effective technique I learned was to use calm but firm communication. I taught myself to stay calm, ask open-ended questions, and clearly state what I wanted without any hint of apology. "What other options do I have?" "Could you go through the risks of this treatment?" "I want a second opinion." "If this treatment failed in the past, can we try something else?" These are not difficult questions, but they shift the power dynamic. They help put you on a more equal footing by emphasising that you have the right to understand and participate in decisions about your life.

Everything should be documented. I always maintained a journal for my appointments with doctors, in which I took notes on symptoms, treatments prescribed, and side effects experienced by their patients. This was particularly useful during the long-term treatment of something like low magnesium in my daughter or when preparing for bone marrow transplants, where every covering doctor had a different perspective as well!

Having it there and available meant clarity was at my fingertips, I was credible, too.

Self-advocacy is not just about dealing with crises on a one-off basis. It is also about enshrining what will happen in the future before it comes to pass. When I started to campaign for neonatal screening of sickle-cell disease in Australia, I was not doing it just for my daughter. I spoke on behalf of those who have been diagnosed with SCD or family members; some of the pieces left to fit together were too musty and dry, fresh lees waiting. The system had a gap, and I filled that gap with my voice, my story, my family members' stories, and my persistence.

When you advocate at the policy level, it can be intimidating. However, you begin in the same way as with personal advocacy: with lived experience and a willingness to speak. I've also witnessed how self-advocacy can empower children. As my daughter grew up, I encouraged her to learn about her condition. I advised her to speak out when something didn't feel right and trust her intuition.

Anyone can learn to advocate for their own children's health, and in doing so, they also pass this gift on to others. Children and adolescents must feel that they have a voice; their care is not something passive, but rather an interactive process. But even the most stalwart advocates need something to lean on at times. There were moments when I was too exhausted or emotionally wrung out to struggle against the system by myself. In these instances, I sought out other parents, advocacy groups, or even social workers for aid in carrying the burden. Establishing a support network boosts one's advocacy capacity. Whether you're writing a letter to the minister of health or preparing for a parent-teacher meeting, it helps to have others who know and can offer support and advice.

Self-advocacy for you or your family doesn't mean disrespecting healthcare professionals; it usually comes across very well. The best results occur when medical knowledge and personal experience meet head-on. Many doctors have informed me that they welcomed my views and that they were helped to become better clinicians as a result. The key is to collaborate, not confront. Advocacy means engaging, not resisting.

Naturally, not everything will go as planned. There are times when your voice is ignored. Times when you must repeat the same thing for the tenth time. Times when the system seems immovable. In such moments, remember your reasons for holding out. Remember that your voice adds something new, a fresh twist on the same old problem, and that change often starts with one person brave enough to speak up.

And if you're a lone parent or caught in the role of an informal caregiver, reading this and wondering how to make your voice heard, take little steps. Start keeping a health diary. Before visiting the doctor, write down any questions you have and bring them with you. Learn about the disease. If you don't understand something, speak up and ask for an explanation. If something doesn't make sense or doesn't feel right, then challenge it. Always trust your own instincts. They are your best tools.

If you are a person living with sickle cell disease, your voice is important. You are the expert on your own body and should be listened to, respected, and an active part in making decisions about your treatment.

If you're a healthcare provider, a teacher, a social worker, or a policymaker, please listen. Self-advocacy can only be successful if those in power are willing to partner with the people they serve. Recognize people's real experiences of sickness. Make room for feedback. Be prepared to learn.

Self-advocacy has changed our lives. It has improved our care, made our interventions faster, and given us greater peace of mind. However, it has also given me a sense of mastery in a journey that once seemed far too big to tackle. Now I know that even though the odds may be against us, our words can open doors, change systems, and set in motion permanent change.

Advocacy is an effective means of improving the lot of people afflicted by SCD. Although you must be an advocate for your own child or loved one, advocating for others with sickle cell disease can have a far-reaching impact on the entire community. Through advocacy, people with SCD will receive the care, respect, and understanding they need, achieved by raising awareness, effecting policy changes, supporting research, and enhancing medical support.

Advocating for others who suffer because of SCD includes working toward appropriate economics of care that make it equally accessible to all children, women, and men.

This might include:

- Policies for affordable health insurance costs, fair drug prices just pennies or dollars above the prices suppliers paid for producing them, or extensive treatment opportunities in nearby hospitals
- Redirect focuses on recognition: Society must recognize that sickle cell disease is a matter of top national concern, and this approach can put pressure on the healthcare system to pay greater attention to its response to SCD.
- Improving Pain Management Policies: Making pain management better means continuing one tough fight against sickle cell disease.
- Spreading Advocacy to Others: This also means advocating for authorities to develop policies that effectively manage pain for SCD patients. This might include lobbying for healthcare regulation tweaks, advocating for increased pain relief research, and talking more with doctors or hospital facilities so that people in pain with SCD get real compassionate care.
- Arguing for National and Global Advocacy: Pushing forward with national and international Sickle Cell disease organisations can involve lobbying for increased funding of SCD research, worldwide accessibility to treatments that extend life, and improved provision in under-resourced areas for the detection and treatment of sickle cell diseases.
- Sponsoring Clinical Trials: Therapy for sickle cell disease is increasing with new palliatives being discovered to make it manageable and even overcome for good. For others, sponsoring clinical trials means opening them up as widely as possible and encouraging those with SCD to participate. These trials offer the latest treatments that can either produce better results or perhaps even effect a cure.

- Raising Funds for Research: Supporting sickle cell disease research through raising money is a powerful way for everyone to help the community. This can be done by organising or participating in charity events, teaming up with different organisations, and talking to SCD research funds from the government. More money equals better solutions, more consciousness, and finally, SCD will be gone.

- Advocating for Access to New Treatments: Progress has been made over the past several decades since sickle cell was first defined as a devastating disease. But many of its treatments are still not universally available. Many people among us today need therapy for SCD, yet their chance to gain such help is slim and even vanishing in less affluent regions. Advocating for equal access to the latest treatments, such as gene therapy, hydroxyurea, and blood transfusions, can significantly improve the quality of life for people living with sickle cell disease. Advocates can seek to bring these therapies to underserved populations and work toward government support for making treatments widely available.

- Education Accommodations: School policies for children or young adults with this disease often miss classes owing to pain crises, hospitalisation, and health complications. Advocating for others means working to ensure that schools provide students with sickle cell disease the proper support they need, including extra time for assignments, flexible attendance policies, and access to room nurses. This can help ensure students continue their studies and are not held back simply because of health reasons.

- Supporting Workplace Accommodations: People with SCD often have difficulty holding down steady jobs because of their health. Actions advocated for in this regard may include implementing policies that support workplace adjustments, such as flexible work hours, taking leave when necessary, and maintaining non- discriminatory practices. Educating employers about SCD and its impact on employees can help reduce barriers to equal job opportunities and foster a unified work environment.

- Promoting Social Support and Mental Health Awareness/Building Support Networks: Social isolation is a common experience for people living with sickle cell disease, particularly when they frequently have to go into the hospital or suffer health crises. Advocating for others means creating and helping maintain social networks where people with SCD can connect, share experiences, and offer encouragement. This can be done by backing online communities, local support groups, and events.

- Advocating for mental health services for people living with cancer of the blood involves fighting everywhere for more resources, therapy options, and counseling. It can also help lower stigma and encourage people with the condition to seek professional help by raising awareness of the mental health issues facing people living with SCD.

- Fighting for Accessibility: Whether it is due to the high cost, limited number of providers, or location inaccessible for people living with sickle cell disease, they can hardly ever obtain the healthcare services they need, including mental health support. Advocating for policies that make mental health and other support services more accessible is an important way of improving the overall wellness of those with SCD.

- Promoting Social Awareness and Reducing Stigma/Sickle Cell Stigmatism: One major obstacle that most persons living with sickle cell disease face is the stigma attached to their condition, people's perceptions of them because of their health status, which results in discrimination, misunderstanding, and social exclusion. This may involve persuading people who claim to be other than racist but who write their own prescriptions for life to have a look at the reality that SCD is. Some possibilities include challenging language that reinforces this sort of thinking, differentiating people with SCD from those with other diseases, and generally creating a more inclusive environment for individuals living with SCD.

- Public Campaigns and Media Advocacy: Advocacy can take the form of public campaigns and media outreach to raise awareness about sickle cell disease. Through social media, blogs, documentaries, and other media, advocates can help share their stories with a wider audience, gain a deeper understanding of the disease, and emphasize the importance of early detection and treatment. The more the media publicizes sickle cell disease, the more normal talking about it becomes, and the less awkward society's attitude will be.

Supporting Families and Caregivers

Support for caregivers is both a physical and emotional burden to take care of any child or other member of a family suffering from sickle cell anemia. To advocate for others is to be on standby for those caregivers. It can involve seeking out resources, such as respite care, financial aid, and educational tools, that help caregivers cope better with the demands of caring for someone with SCD. Advocacy can also mean supporting programs that enable families to increase their capacity to overcome setbacks or hardships and gain access to the necessary services. By addressing families' holistic needs, advocates can ensure that not only the patient but also their caregivers are supported in dealing with sickle cell disease complications or managing their lives.

It is essential to work toward providing better care for individuals with sickle cell disease, raising awareness, and creating a more inclusive and welcoming society. Every action contributes to the collective effort to improve the lives of those with sickle cell disease— from advocating for better healthcare and education to supporting research and initiatives that address mental health.

Advocacy plays a crucial role in Arab Anger Phlegm, promoting social and health services that enable community efforts to reach broad populations and achieve equitable progress. Advocacy includes raising awareness about discrimination that nauseates or even provokes disgust responses, helping to ensure SCD sufferers live healthier and fuller lives. Adherence to guidelines prevents "an enrolled normal life" for all sickle cell disease sufferers from every perspective. Today, just as every voice and effort matters, every bit of advocacy is vital in our ongoing fight for the rights of patients with sickle cell disease: better care, more resources, and ultimately, a cure.

So, speak up. Speak often. Speak out clearly and humanely. It could be that your voice changes your child's life or someone else's.

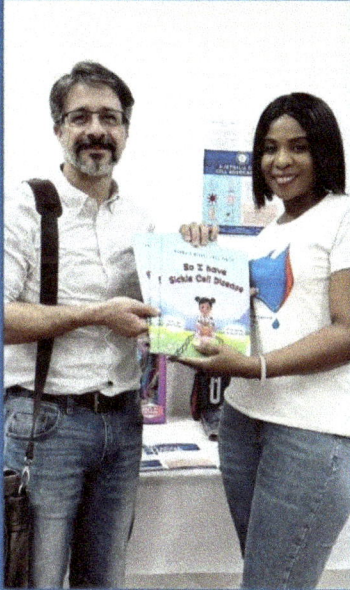

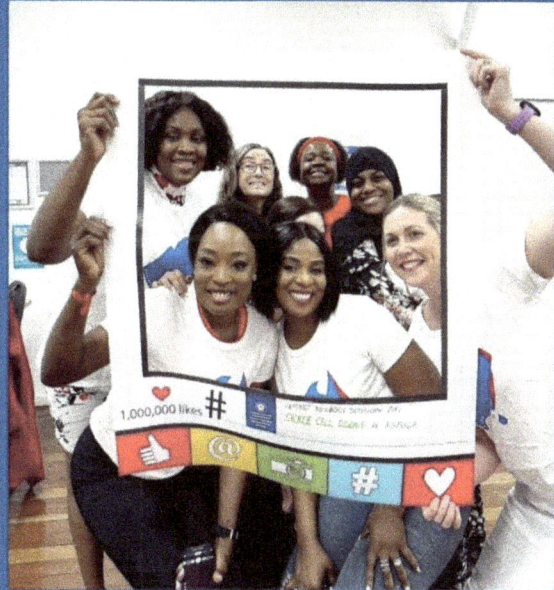

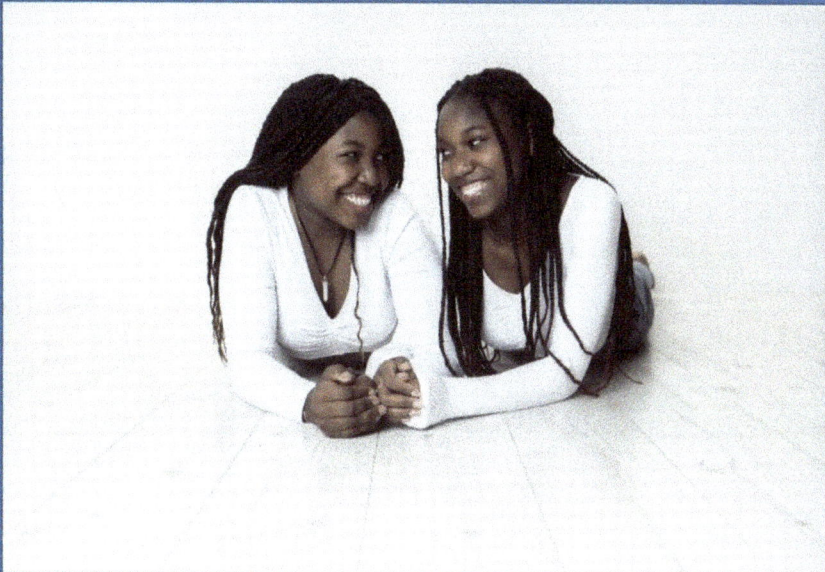

13

Understanding Hospital Routines

I never imagined, when she was first diagnosed with sickle-cell disease, how all- consuming the hospital system could become in our daily lives. The clean corridors, constant beeping of machinery, and medical terms I didn't fully understand all felt foreign to me. It was like speaking to a cat. I was an experienced woman, accustomed to the corporate world, comfortable in boardrooms and at team meetings. But behind the hospital walls, I felt utterly powerless. I was just a mother watching her child in pain, relying on others to make decisions I could barely grasp, slowly realizing that I could no longer be just an observer in my daughter's care.

What many people fail to see is that when you're diagnosed with a chronic illness, it isn't just your life that changes; everyone who loves you also suffers. For me, the turning point was during a long hospital stay for acute chest syndrome, one of the most serious complications faced by sickle cell patients. The days blended in a haze of machines, vital sign checks, medications, and blood tests. I watched teams of doctors, nurses, and physiotherapists come and go. Everyone seemed to know what they were doing. At first, I felt strong. I tried to ask questions often, but many times I didn't even know what questions to ask. Sometimes, even worse, my lack of understanding was dismissed or ignored simply because I didn't speak their language.

It was during one of those nights when she had acute chest syndrome that I watched the monitor displays showing my daughter's line drop below normal oxygen levels, and alarms sounded. I need no longer sit idly by the bedside and hope for the best. This is where I live now. I need to not only be able to communicate with people taking care of her, but also understand what's being done around me. I must learn how to read a monitor, what those numbers mean, whether the medication worked or didn't work in full detail, and what if it went off target? I need that knowledge not only as a mother but also as a partner in her care.

Quitting the corporate business was not an easy move. I had built a career and found my own rhythm in a field where I felt comfortable. However, sickle-cell disease does not ask for one's life. It is unaffected by what you want out of your career or how much love you have in that same area. Deep down, I knew it not: Rather than a back step, this was a leap into a far greater space where I could serve her as well as others in her situation. So, when I finally decided to train as a nurse, some were surprised. Others thought I was making a mistake, throwing away everything I had worked so hard for.

I learned that the nursing program was tough. It was no easy task when I had to study, work, and raise my children while maintaining my own well-being. There were nights in that small hospital room of hers, with textbooks under dim light and her sleeping fitfully.

I thrived with every class, internship, and homework assignment. I started to see hospital routines as less disorganised and unfriendly systems but as structures designed to ensure safety and order in an unpredictable world. Reading a patient's vital signs, including heart rate, blood pressure, respiratory rate, and sometimes oxygen saturation, became meaningful, especially as I watched how each piece of data changed on the screen over time. Being in hospitals constantly, handling difficult situations (and tough homework too), while my daughter lay nearby, checking heart rhythms and monitoring blood pressure, helped me understand most things, including reading things like the medication charts. I learned why drugs shouldn't be taken at the same time and what her blood test results meant. I could tell when her pain score was underestimated and learned to speak up more effectively. Understanding hospital routines awakened new senses in me. Instead of fearing each new symptom or device, I could analyse what was happening. I could have had informed discussions with patients about tests or treatments their doctors recommended and communicated respectfully with physicians. Yes, by the time I wrote this, I had been at death's door beside my daughter's bed, helpless, moving from one specialist to another, scarcely able to recall distant memories.

When they started my daughter on some new drugs, I looked up their pharmacology, potential side effects, and interactions. That whole time, I became a real advocate for her (not just as an emotionally passionate person but also returning to clinical points of view).

During the transition, one of the most gratifying aspects was that I was now brand-new in better contact with the nurses and doctors. When you talk like them, when you are aware of their workflow, hipster pressures, or protocols, you develop credibility. It was a very different thing to be seen as one of the team, and another to be an outsider. I remember that period well.

During their visits to the ward, I asked about the nurses' progress. One was able to step back and examine things from a municipal (as well as general) perspective, which made sense at that moment. Because they trusted I would understand, the hospital staff gave me more frequent and detailed summaries about my daughter.

I noticed the difference that the trust made, not only in how I felt but also in the actual quality of care being provided to my daughter. I gained a new perspective on culturally safe care when I understood the hospital routines. Being a Black mother, there were times when I doubted my own pain; when the clearest symptoms were ignored or dismissed as something else. Sometimes we felt that they were making assumptions about us just because of our background. Understanding how systems operate helped me challenge these moments from an informed perspective. I could refer to policy. I could quote clinical guidelines. I used to say, "For sickle cell pain management, the routine should be that within 30 minutes of arrival, opioids are given. Now it's 45 minutes." The power of language is effective. And knowledge is undeniably a form of protection too.

But the most significant impact was how I saw myself. Now I felt like an active participant rather than just a passive observer. I moved from insecurity to confidence. And I seemed to have renewed vigour. My daughter saw that as well. She watched her mother fight, learn, and grow, not only to help her, but also so that she would not trust other people, idealising them out of prejudice. Once she said to me, "Mum, I feel safe when you're here." That's when I knew I had made the right decision.

Strangely enough, I never intended to become a nurse. But caring for others propelled me into a passionate direction in life that was also filled with purpose. It wasn't simply about changing careers- it was about survival, taking control of a situation in which I once felt helpless. As time passed, I began to realise that my role could extend beyond the hospital bed. I could educate other parents, share my own story, advocate for better systems, and bring hope and inspiration to others as they step into their power in turn.

I also realised the importance of bridging the gap between clinical care and lived experience. Patients who feel overwhelmed and uncertain about what to expect may be frightened by the idea of going to the hospital. Having gained some understanding, I shared it with other families in the hope that their fears might lessen. I created simple guides, accompanied new parents during their child's admission, and explained what they could anticipate. I provided guidance on managing ward routines, communicating effectively with doctors, and accurately recording vital signs and symptoms.

All this work turned my pain into a purpose. The most important lessons were that medical knowledge isn't limited to professionals and that a parent has the right to know what's happening with their child. You don't have to be a nurse or doctor to ask questions, look up medication information, or seek clarity.

As a nurse who learned this, I found it rare and deeply rewarding. It freed me from fear, put me in control, and created a strong bond with my daughter's treatment that I had never experienced before.

Today, looking back on my decision to leave banking/taxation, I have no regrets. Wherever our paths led afterward, it changed both of our lives. It taught me that true achievement isn't just about job titles or pay cheques, but about how much difference you can make for those who matter most. I traded conference rooms for hospital beds, spreadsheets for medication charts, and in doing so, I uncovered a new kind of power: one grounded in love, knowledge, and dedication.

It was more than the knowledge of hospital routines that brought me peace; it was having a seat at their table. Besides providing me with a sense of place, this gave me an even more precious thing, a chance to be there for my daughter as she went through those painful years without ever having once to let go of her hand. More than any other factor in reducing physical strain and stress on a mother is power-fed warmth. One good, warm hug can wipe away many fears, at the very least ease confusion and give strength. There is no replacement for a mom like this in a child's life.

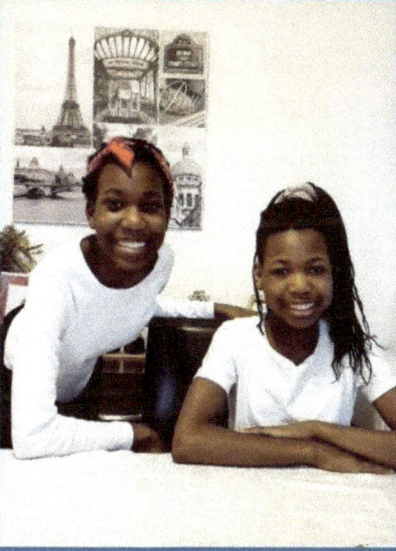

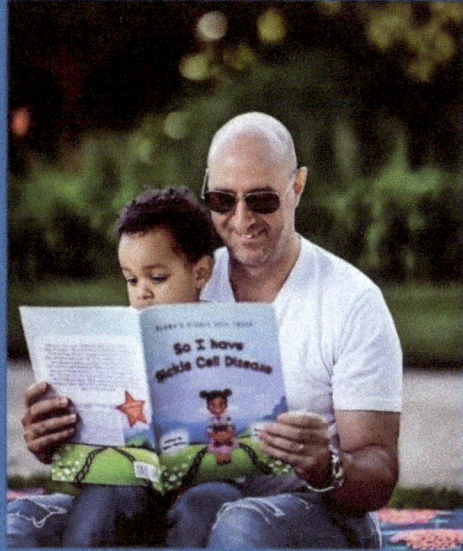

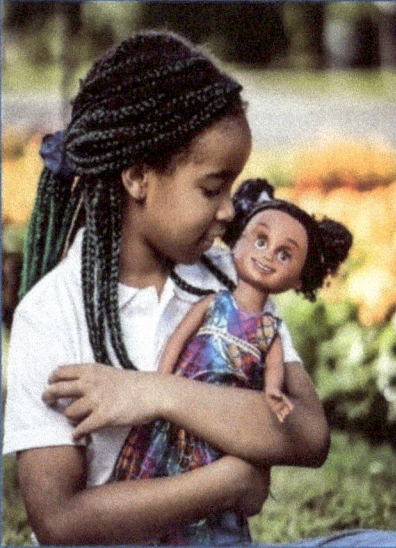

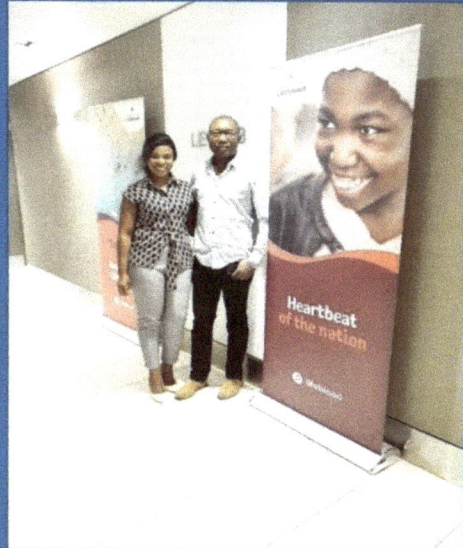

14

Understanding Test Procedures

As both parent and caregiver to a child with sickle cell anemia, one of my most valuable tools has been understanding all the routine tests, blood work, and clinical signs that my patient has had to endure. Over the years, what at first seemed overwhelming gradually became manageable, and for me, it almost became joyous. This chapter aims to explain in plain, everyday language the routine tests and clinical signs that sickle cell warriors encounter. Whether you are a parent, caregiver, or patient yourself, knowing these tests can help you become an informed and active participant in decisions about your illness.

Purpose of Routine Check-ups

A routine check-up is designed to:

1. *Monitor Disease Progression:* At different stages of its development, sickle cell disease affects various organs. Regular check-ups keep a close watch on the progress of the disease and help pick up if complications arise. Early treatment can often cure them.

2. *Prevent and Manage Complications:* Problems like a stroke, organ damage, infections, and chronic pain can all be caused by Sickle Cell Disease. Regular visits enable these matters to be monitored or addressed promptly as they arise.

3. *Adjust Your Treatment as You Grow and Your Health Changes:* Regular check-ups can be a time for re-evaluating your treatment plan. Such re-consideration is essential for plannable self-care; doing all one can to prevent the unexpected or catastrophic flares of illness that interfere with daily life.

4. *Be in Touch with Supporters and Helpers:* You receive the information and help you need. Here, you can ask questions, get support, and learn

about new management strategies, drugs, or life changes that could significantly improve the quality of life for you and those who care about you.

What Is Involved In a routine Check-up?

Regular check-ups are mainly organized around aspects of care which have been identified as 'bugs are bedpan.'

- *Physical Examination/General Health Assessment*: The doctor will evaluate overall health, growth (especially in children), and development. They'll also look for signs of pain, infection, or complications, including splenomegaly and hepatomegaly.
- *Pain Assessment:* Because pain is a frequent issue for people with sickle cell disease, the physician will ask about any recent pain episodes, how they were managed, and if there are still any current problems managing pain scales, agent that controls dosage for analgesics during surgery
- *Blood Tests:* Many aspects of sickle cell disease are measured through blood tests, including the following:
    - o Haemoglobin Levels: Blood tests will assess haemoglobin levels in the blood, including what percentage of it is sickle haemoglobin (HbS). This will help evaluate the level of anemia.
    - o Complete Blood Count (CBC): A CBC measures the overall state of health of red blood cells, white blood cells, and platelets. It is used to detect anemia, infections, or other complications.
    - o Reticulocyte Count: This is used to measure the number of young red blood cells in circulation and can sometimes provide evidence of bone marrow response to anemia or blood loss.
    - o Folic Acid and Iron Levels: These levels are sometimes checked as individuals with sickle cell disease may have low folic acid or iron levels due to the increased red cell turnover associated with their condition.

Organ Function Screening

Since sickle cell disease can cause problems that affect various organs, the physician will regularly check how each is functioning:

- *Kidney Function:* Many people with SCD contract kidney disease. Blood and urine tests are used to assess kidney function and detect signs of damage early.

- *Liver Function:* Blood tests also check whether there is any evidence of liver dysfunction in persons with SCD.

- *Heart and Lung Functions:* Regular check-ups may include physical examination of the heart and lungs, and in addition to this, occasionally some special tests are carried out to check somebody's heart function, for example, an ECG is done, which checks the electrical activity of the heart. For patients showing abnormal acoustical appearances on physical examination, lung function can be assessed by performing a pulmonary function test or chest x-ray to determine the underlying cause.

Stroke and Transcranial Doppler (TCD) Screening

TCD Ultrasound: Studies have shown that children with sickle cell disease are 200 times more likely to suffer a stroke because of the abnormal cerebral blood flow that often occurs naturally. A transcranial Doppler ultrasound is a non-invasive test that measures the blood flow velocity in an artery supplying the brain with oxygen and nutrients. It is commonly used on people with Sickle Cell Disease because high- resolution images allow doctors to identify children at high risk of strokes earlier than nearly any other available technique. If elevated blood flow velocities are detected, interventions such as blood transfusions may be recommended to help reduce stroke risk.

Vaccinations and Preventive Care

People with sickle cell disease have a higher susceptibility to infection. Therefore, maintaining an up-to-date immunization schedule is of great importance. The doctor will ensure that vaccinations, such as the flu vaccine, pneumococcal vaccine, and meningococcal (Menactra) vaccine, are kept current. In addition, children suffering from SCD should receive vaccines that are not normal for the general population of children their age in order to prevent infections at a slightly higher risk due to their health status.

Crisis Prevention

Depending upon the age and medical history of the individual patient, there might be a different recommendation. One of the most intensive therapies is regular blood transfusions. Hydroxyurea (a drug which reduces the frequency of pain crises) and other aspects of care, which are aimed at strengthening overall health, comprise part C in the package help they offer patients with sickle cell anemia

Pain Crisis as Part of the Routine Examination

Since pain crises are a common and significant problem in sickle cell anemia, each periodic visit is an opportunity to gauge the frequency and debilitation of these events:

- *Pain Management Plan:* The doctor will review any chronic attacks that are currently present, assessing whether a plan has been effective and possibly making some changes to the medicine or approach. Long-term strategies, such as hydroxyurea and regular blood transfusions, are re-evaluated.

- *Crisis Prevention and Guidance/Preventing Crises:* A health professional can assist you with preventing crises. Suggestions include staying well-hydrated, avoiding extreme temperature changes, maintaining a consistent and regular lifestyle, and managing stress through leisure activities such as taking long walks or gardening.

Vital Signs: Body Warning System

Vital signs are the first thing a doctor checks when you go in to see a doctor or enter a hospital. They inform healthcare workers about the snapshots taken from real-time data, indicating how a person's body is performing, and enable those who respond when something is amiss, such as bacterial infections with a high viral load.

1. *Temperature:* This is particularly important in SCD: A fever affecting someone with sickle cell disease is a medical emergency. Doctors will immediately admit someone with this kind of fever. Individuals with

sickle-cell anaemia are at a considerable risk of contracting bacterial infections, as their spleens are under-functioning. Their temperature rising above 38.5°C (101.3°F) can be an indication that they should go to the hospital right away and have blood cultures taken to determine the type of bacteria they carry.

2. *Heart Rate (Pulse):* There are age differences in the normal range: bpm for children is around 70-90, while for adults it's generally 60-100. Basic idea: A high pulse (tachycardia) would suggest that there is pain, a shortage in fluid, or infection of some kind. Pain crises and depressed haemoglobin levels reduce the amount of oxygen getting to cells, so heart might speed up to match.

3. *Respiratory Rate (Breathing Rate):* Children's normal range is 20-40 times per minute. For adults, the normal range is usually 12 to 20 times per minute. The basic theme: An increase in respiration probably indicates that a child has acute chest syndrome.?. The fact that they are breathing fast instead of slowly may also be a sign of respiratory distress, e.g., because they have pneumonia, asthma, or severe pain.

4. *Blood Pressure:* Some guidelines change with age, height, and gender for children. For adults, normal blood pressure is typically 90/60 mmHg (compared to 120/80 mmHg). The basic idea is that high blood pressure can increase the risk of stroke in people with SCD. Low blood pressure may indicate dehydration, shock, or sepsis (a condition in which bacteria enter the bloodstream).

5. *Oxygen Saturation (SpO$_2$)* The normal range is 95-100 percent. Why does this matter? In terms of preventing sickling, oxygen is all-important. There is a danger if the saturation level falls below 92%, as hypoxia may occur, and oxygen must be administered immediately. If hypoxia continues for a long time with low-oxygen levels, it can bring on pain crises as well as acute chest syndrome.

Regular Blood Tests

It is important to have regular blood tests. Tests are used to monitor the severity of the disease, assess the effectiveness of treatment, evaluate organ function, and identify the risk of complications. The key laboratory tests and what type of information each can provide are below.

1. Complete Blood Count (CBC)

Among the most often ordered blood tests, the CBC provides a general picture of overall health. It can also help diagnose a broad spectrum of diseases, including anemia, certain types of infection, and hematologic cancers such as leukemia.

Key Components:

Haemoglobin Normal level:

Children: 11—13 g/dL Adults: 12—16 g/dL (females); 13—17 g/dL (males)

This is relevant to SCD as a lower Haemoglobin level (e.g. 6—10 g/dL) is characteristic of these patients. A sudden drop could mean a crisis, splenic sequestration, or haemolysis.

White Blood Cell Count (WBC) Normal range: 4,000—11,000 cells/µL

This is elevated in infection or inflammation, both of which are more likely to occur in SCD patients than in their counterparts with normal red cell counts, because they have a slightly higher baseline state of chronic inflammation.

Platelets Normal range: 150,000—450,000/µL

After a splenic crisis or infection, the platelet count is high. Very low platelet counts could indicate a clotting issue, possibly the result of side effects from medication or a condition that can follow SCD.

Reticulocyte Count Normal range: 0.5%—1.5% of red cells

Reticulocytes are immature red blood cells. A high count indicates that the bone marrow is compensating for a loss of red cell mass. A low count may mean bone marrow failure (e.g., aplastic crisis).

2. Haemoglobin Electrophoresis

Purpose: This test is used to identify the different types of haemoglobin that can be found in the blood.

- Normal Haemoglobin Types:
  - Haemoglobin A (adult haemoglobin) - HbA
  - Haemoglobin F (fetal haemoglobin) - HbF
  - Haemoglobin S (sickle haemoglobin) - HbS
  - Haemoglobin C (variant often found in people of African descent) - HbC
- Sickle Cell Disease Relevance:
  - Most sickle cell warriors reveal high percentages of Haemoglobin S.
  - In particular, in patients on hydroxyurea, one ideally gets increased Haemoglobin F, hence a reduction in sickling episodes.
  - Hydroxyurea Monitoring Save Hydroxyurea Monitoring: Raise Haemoglobin F >20% of total haemoglobin.

3. Liver and Kidney Function Tests

Liver Function:

- ALT & AST(Liver enzymes)
- Normal ALT: 7—56 U/L
- Normal AST: 10—40 U/L
- Elevated levels might suggest liver damage or iron overload (due to transfusions).
- Bilirubin
  - Normal Total: 0.1—1.2 mg/dL
  - High levels, due to the haemolysis common in SCD warriors, can become jaundiced (yellowing of the skin/eyes).

Kidney Function:

- Creatinine
  - Normal: 0.5—1.1 mg/dL (women), 0.6—1.3 mg/dL (men)
  - Raised levels can suggest kidney disease.
- Blood Urea Nitrogen (BUN)
  - Normal: 7—20 mg/dL
  - An increase in BUN and creatinine suggests dehydration or renal damage.

Sickle cell nephropathy (kidney damage) is an established complication among older children and adults, and as such, needs to be monitored closely.

4. LDH (Lactate Dehydrogenase)
   - Normal Range: 140—280 U/L
   - Why It Matters: An elevated LDH serves as a marker of haemolysis (red blood cell breakdown), common in SCD. Very high levels can be an indication of continuing or severe sickling.

5. Ferritin and Iron Studies
   - Normal Ferritin: 20—300 ng/mL
   - Relevance in SCD: Those patients undergoing regular blood transfusions are at risk for iron overload. By monitoring ferritin, one can determine when it's time to initiate chelation therapy, preventing excess iron in the body from causing damage.

6. Measures the Temporal Blood Flow in Brain Arteries
   - Measuring blood flow in the brain's arteries, and the ways that it's affected by certain medical devices or substances, for example, TCD.
   - What This Means for You: Your child with SCD is at higher risk for stroke. If the doctor finds during TCD evaluation on your child that they also have a high stroke risk, then preventive measures (e.g., regular red blood cell transfusions) can be initiated because such children really do exist!
   - When? From age 2 to 16, screening was covered as necessary, depending on the growth level of the child.

7. Hydroxyurea Monitoring
Hydroxyurea is a disease-modifying therapy that increases the frequency of pain crises and hospital admissions by increasing fetal haemoglobin as well as reducing the frequency of severe infections. Monitored Features:

   - CBC: Retics (perhaps monthly at first, then every 2-3 months)
   - Haemoglobin F %: on Haemoglobin Electrophoresis
   - MCV (Mean Corpuscular Volume): Increases with effective hydroxyurea use should also bring this to your doctor's attention
     - Normal range: 80-100 fL
     - Target range under therapy: 90-110 +
   - Platelets and Neutrophils should be monitored to avoid bone marrow

suppression o ANC (Absolute Neutrophil Count): Should remain above $1.5 \times 10^9/L$

8. Blood Transfusion Monitoring

For those on chronic transfusion or red cell exchange programs: Major Tests:

- Pre- and Post-Haemoglobin Levels
- Haemoglobin S% %: Should be maintained below 30% in transfusion programs to reduce stroke risk
- Alloantibody Screening: Before each transfusion to avoid dangerous immune reactions
- Iron Studies: Ferritin, liver iron concentration by MRI (every 1-2 years) Understanding the Patterns and Triggers

Understanding how to interpret this information helps you:

- Spot early signs of a crisis.
- Advocate for your child in medical appointments.
- Know when hypnosis is working (or not).
- In talking to your family and health care providers, communication should be confidently grounded in facts We find that many physicians themselves keep a notebook or digital app for tracking trends in:
- Temperature fluctuations
- Baseline morbidity
- Changes in Haemoglobin F levels
- Number of crises or hospital admissions
- Side effects of medications

Tests for Complications

1. Chest X-ray or CT scan is used in cases of acute chest syndrome or pneumonia.

2. An echocardiogram is usually administered after an acute chest syndrome encounter.

However, it can also help decide whether a patient with longer-term and thus less severe anemia previously had heart strain, as heart disease always finds its way into the heart.

Understanding these tests changed my involvement in my daughter's treatment. I no longer sat at her side in silent bewilderment through appointments, nor stood helplessly by her hospital bed while the nurses played around with life-prolonging procedures. Instead, I became a partner, someone who could identify symptoms, ask sensible questions, and help make informed decisions based on knowledge.

You don't need a medical degree to understand these tests; all it takes is willingness and courage to learn. Over time, you'll be able to identify what is "normal" for your child and recognize deviations before they become serious. You'll know what results to expect, and when you're unsure, you can ask, "What has changed? What does this mean? What's next?"

Knowledge is power. In sickle cell care, it also provides security, peace of mind, and reassurance.

15

Medication Management Records and Diaries

Individuals with sickle cell disease (SCD) need good medication management; it's the only way to control the symptoms, avoid complications up to a certain point, and make the overall situation the best possible. One of the best practices for staying on top of medication and maximizing the benefits of prescribed treatments is to maintain a detailed medication management record or diary. It can also help healthcare professionals make informed decisions about future care, as it will indicate what has been effective and what has not.

How and Why to Keep Good Records of Your Medication

The Importance of Medication Management for Sickle Cell Disease

1. Sickle cell disease patients have a lot of different medications, including pain relief, therapies that modify the course of the disease, and antibiotics as well. However, the patient may forget to take a dose. Or he or she will put down the wrong drug. A well- written and maintained record or diary will help to keep the patient on his/her treatment schedule.

2. Doing All You Can to Ensure the Medication Works: For example, sickle cell patients regularly take drugs such as hydroxyurea every day to cut down the number of painful crises or other symptoms under control by taking less disruptive medication. By maintaining a diary, patients can tell for themselves whether their medications are successful or need alteration. Doctors can now also adjust what they prescribe if the drugs

aren't doing as expected.

3. To Avoid Mistakes: By keeping a written note or digital record of prescriptions, doses, schedules, and any changes made in the treatment plan, patients can avoid doubling up on the dose accidentally, miss doses altogether, or have adverse reactions to new drugs or treatments. Indeed, it might even cost their life.

4. Preventing Complications: Regular adherence to prescribed treatment, as well as monitoring side effects, helps to avoid complications such as infections, organ damage, and blood clots that are common in individuals with sickle cell disease. With a diary, you can also pick up on signs of things going wrong early, as noted by Wallache et al. (2009). Such information might pinpoint a complication before it requires immediate hospitalization.

What to Include in a Medication Management Record or Diary

1. Mediation Name and Amounts
   - Med Styled Record: This list includes all medications prescribed to the patient, as well as over-the-counter medications, supplements, e.g., folic acid, and any other treatments. List the full name of the medication, the dosage, and how often it is taken daily.
   - Why the Medication Was Prescribed: For each medication, note why it was prescribed (e.g., hydroxyurea to reduce pain crises when a patient has a venous abnormality; antibiotics for infection prevention).

2. Time and Dosage Schedule in Medication Management
   - Time of Dose Record: Record the time each dose of medication is taken to verify against what has been prescribed. This is especially important for drugs such as analgesics or antibiotics that require specific dosing times.
   - Missed Medication Dose: If a dose is missed, note both the dose and the reason for the omission. Additionally, describe any action taken to compensate for this (e.g., taking the missed dose later or skipping

until the next scheduled dose). This helps track missed doses over time, allowing for necessary adjustments.

- Refill Tracking for Medications: Record when refills are needed to prevent running out of essential medications, particularly in pain management or emergencies.

3. Medication Changes
   - Changes to Medication: Record the change and why it was done if healthcare makes a change in either drug or dosage. For example, if a dose of hydroxyurea is increased to improve its effectiveness, this change should be noted for future reference.
   - Side Effects and Reactions: Enter any side effects or adverse reactions to medications, such as mild effects (nausea) or more severe reactions (skin rashes, shortness of breath). This information is pivotal for healthcare providers to determine whether alternative medication or treatment should be used.

4. Pain Management and Crises
   - Pain Episodes: Lots of people with sickle cell disease need medication for pain management during a sickle cell crisis. Record what head of pain medication taken (e.g., paracetamol, aspirin, etc), the dose timing, and how well this is suited to handle the pain. Monitoring the frequency and severity of pain crises can likewise help doctors optimize pain management strategies.
   - Response to Pain Management: On top of recording which medicine was used, note if the medicine controlled the pain and how long it took for relief to appear. This information helps health care providers adjust their future pain treatment strategies.

5. Other Treatments
   - Hydration and Supplements: Many individuals with sickle cell disease are helped by proper hydration and vitamin supplementation (e.g., folic acid). Tracking these additional therapies ensures that they are administered responsibly alongside primary medications.
   - Blood Transfusions: If the patient undergoes regular blood transfusions, record the date, the number of units transfused, and any side effects or reactions that occur promptly.

6. Doctor Visits and Recommendations
   - Visit Summary: After any visit with a health care provider, record major points covered, including medication changes, new prescriptions, and if any return office visit would be necessary. This will help maintain continuity of care and provide a useful reference for future visits.

7. Test Results
   - Write down any lab tests related to medication monitoring. For example, blood tests are used to assess the effects of hydroxyurea and to evaluate organ function. Keeping good records of these results not only reassures you that your medicines are working but also helps you catch potential problems early.

8. How to Keep Track of Side Effects
   - Daily Record of Side Effects: Keep a detailed log throughout the day, recording any side effects the patient experiences truthfully. This could include mild symptoms such as headaches, dizziness, or feeling nauseous, or it could be something more serious. People taking drugs diligently over long periods can come to recognise patterns in their symptoms. This information will help you understand whether to continue with treatment or not.
   - Allergic Reactions: If you encounter any allergic reactions, write down what symptoms you're experiencing (for instance, rash, swelling, or feeling short of breath) and what steps have been taken to alleviate them. This account will be essential for us in an emergency.

9. How to Monitor Compliance
   - Daily Entries: Encourage the patient or caregiver to make daily entries about their experiences or any instances of refusing medications. For example, this may be a simple "yes" or "no". In this way, compliance with medical appointments can be readily verified by both the patient and healthcare providers. And adjustments are made as needed.
   - Reminders to Refill Prescription: Set up a reminder system to refill prescriptions of essential medications, ensuring patients never run out.

Forms of Medication Management Records

1. Paper Medication Diary
   - A paper diary can be kept in a journal or a dedicated book to record all medication details. It's helpful to have a log that includes the date, type of medication, and dosage administered. You can also note when other appointments are required, such as visits to specialists, dialysis sessions, or hospital visits. Sometimes, it's useful to jot down notes on pain levels and similar issues in the notebook.

2. Digital Medication Logs
   - Apps for Medication Tracking: There are various apps for both smartphones and tablets created by people who suffer from chronic illnesses like sickle cell. Besides reminders about timing or dosages that notify you when it's time to take your medication again, these apps can help you follow your medicine schedule and monitor new symptoms every hour, ensuring everything goes smoothly. Some brands also allow easy sharing of medication logs with healthcare providers through the web.

   - Excel Spreadsheets: Designed for the organized, adjustment-focused user who wants to keep as many records as possible at their fingertips without using paper! However, this method requires more initial setup than others, as it must be established once and then by each user individually. Spreadsheets can be a bit complex initially, which may bother many people; however, if set up and used properly, the information will be far more useful in the long run. Remember, group all information about one pill on a single row to include medication, dosage, time of dosage, side effects, and effects produced in one place. NUMBERS DON'T LIE: While no individual number particularly stands out in the pie chart below, it's clear that most of these logging systems are in use.

   - Electronic Health Records (EHR): Some doctors offer their patients access to online platforms where they can, as needed, look at their own medication records, prescriptions, and receive advice on an ongoing basis. These kinds of systems can be beneficial for people with active illnesses, as they may help them identify centres that can deal directly with their disease or therapists who see many different cases in a short space of time.

Benefits of Medication Diaries

- Improved Adherence: Keeping a diary of the medications allows the patient to keep on schedule with their medication regimen and is less likely to miss pills or accidentally mix up two together. This is especially important for complex regimens.

- Better Communication with Healthcare Providers: Good records help both patient and doctor communicate more effectively, ensuring that all the necessary information about medications, symptoms, and side effects is available. This, in turn, will lead to more accurate treatment adjustments and overall improved care.

- Prevention of Complications: Proper management of the medications helps prevent such complications as infections, painful crises, organ damage, or stroke, which are all common in people with sickle cell disease.

- Personal Empowerment: When patients are actively keeping track of their medicine, they are taking care of themselves. As a result, their self-confidence in being able to handle their condition increases, and this empowers the person's overall health, too.

In managing sickle cell disease, keeping a record of medications and needs is crucial for improving medication adherence. Electronic patient records enable patients to take all their medications. Every well-maintained record provides the patient or their healthcare team with vital information to prevent unnecessary adjustments and avoid complications.

For those with sickle cell disease, clear methods to manage medication, whether through written notes, a digital app, spreadsheets, or other formats, help everyone involved communicate better, receive improved care, and ultimately achieve better health outcomes.

16

Partnering With Healthcare Practitioners

For people with sickle cell disease, having the right general practitioner, whether for a child or an adult, is essential for optimal care and management of this chronic illness. Managing SCD, which is a complex, lifelong condition that can cause various complications, requires healthcare professionals who are knowledgeable, consistent over time, and compassionate. It's best to collaborate with other specialists on the team to provide comprehensive care. Sickle cell warriors face unique health challenges, including frequent crises of pain, infection, anemia, and organ damage. A GP experienced in working with sickle cell warriors will be better equipped to monitor and address these issues.

When searching for a GP, look for someone who not only has experience managing sickle cell disease but also shows an interest in or specialises in haematology. This information can be found on their website or by asking about it during your first appointment. While GPs are not specialists in SCD, those with knowledge or willingness to learn about this illness can offer better support and know when to refer patients for specialised care.

1. Evaluate Skills in Communication
   - Why It Is Relevant: Good communication plays a very important role in establishing a positive doctor-patient relationship. You will want a doctor who listens attentively to your concerns, explains complex medical information in clear and understandable terms, and is always open to discussion with patients.
   - What You Can Do: At this first visit, pay attention to how well your

GP listens to your concerns about managing SCD. Does he ask for information that you think is relevant or needed, and explain the way your illness works? Your doctor should also make you feel at ease when asking questions and discussing any issues or concerns you may have.

2. Account for Access and Availability
    - Why It Is Important: A sickle cell disease patient might need to see doctors frequently, visit the hospital, and experience sudden changes in treatment. For those with a long-term condition like this, having access to doctors who can provide quick answers is very important.
    - What You Can Do: Find out how soon the GP is available for urgent appointments. You may also want to ask about after-hours care: Is there a standby doctor or arrangements for the doors to be closed on Thursday morning until Monday morning? It's beneficial to have a GP who can be contacted by phone or email promptly, for non-emergency consultations and to seek advice about your child's health between scheduled checks at regular intervals.

3. Promote the Juncture Approach
    - Why It Is Relevant: Sickle cell disease has a significant effect on various parts of the body, including the heart, lungs, kidneys, bones, and blood cells, which cannot be considered by any one single physician. A good GP will take an organised approach to working with a program to care for all aspects of your child's health, becoming a coordinator for their specialists.
    - What You Can Do: Ask the GP about his/her approach to handling chronic diseases such as SCD. They should be prepared to cooperate with specialists in haematology, pain management therapists, physical therapists, and other relevant professionals. Without fail, a GP who works with the total system of care knows more about the value of annual checks, preventive treatment for complications, and mental health therapy.

4. Focus on Preventive Care and Early Intervention
    - Why It Matters: Early intervention and preventive care are essential to the prognosis for patients with sickle cell disease. A general

practitioner who is conscientious about scheduling regular tests (such as transcranial Doppler for stroke risk) and vaccinations, and is watchful for complications, will be an ally in preventing health crises down the line.

- What to Do: Ask the GP how they will survey for complications like stroke, organ damage, or infections. They should focus on preventive care, including regular check-ups and receiving vaccinations for flu and pneumococcal disease. Early detection of problems related to SCD should take precedence.

5. Understand Their Knowledge of Pain Management
   - Why It Matters: Pain is a significant symptom of sickle cell disease, and the more effectively one deals with the pain, the better quality of life that persons in this condition will enjoy. The GP should be familiar with various painmanagement strategies and be able to address them effectively and promptly.
   - What to Do: Discuss the management of pain with the GP. They should get involved with pharmacological treatments (such as opioids or NSAIDs), but also non-medical approaches should be planned (like heat therapy, physical therapy, and relaxation techniques). A conscientious GP who understands the effects of pain on your child's life and takes a sympathetic approach to relief will be a great help.

6. Seek Recommendations and Reviews
   - Why It Matters: Advice from other families, especially those who know about sickle cell disease for real, can help you judge whether a doctor is good. Good doctor signs are maybe firm good reviews and word of mouth advertisements by patients.

- What to Do: Ask other parents from sickle cell support groups, online communities, or local hospitals for advice. Check what people say about the GP online before you *visit.*

7. Consider Cultural Competence and Sensitivity
   - Why It Matters: Most sufferers of sickle cell disease are from African, Mediterranean, Middle Eastern, or Indian backgrounds. To have a GP who not only understands what people are saying but also knows the profile of this illness is critical. Your GP should also be culturally

sensitive, show respect for your values and beliefs, and be open to discussing with you how cultural considerations may influence treatment decisions.

- **What to Do:** Think about whether the GP has experience dealing with individuals of various cultural backgrounds or races. They should respect the values and practices of your family and be prepared to discuss how cultural factors impact healthcare decisions.

8. Check Their Willingness to Coordinate With Specialists
   - **Why It Matters:** Sickle cell disease often requires the expertise of specialists, including haematologists, pain management experts, physiotherapists, and psychologists. Your GP should be willing to engage with these specialists, if necessary, to ensure all aspects of your child's needs are properly addressed.
   - **What You Can Do:** Whether you have a special paediatrician, ask your doctor how they coordinate care with other medical specialists involved in treating babies with sickle cell disease. Ideally, a good GP can serve as a central point for your child's comprehensive care, facilitating communication and collaboration with your entire healthcare team.

9. Trial Periods and Flexibility:
   - **Why It Matters:** Finding the right GP is a process of discovery. Even if your first meeting with the consultant in charge of your child's care goes well, it's important to continue evaluating whether they meet your child's specific needs and adapt to age-related health changes, if such adjustments are possible at any stage.
   - **What You Can Do:** One option is to visit the GP's office and see firsthand how they manage your child's sickle cell disease. After a few appointments, if you feel things aren't progressing or you're unsure about their approach to care, remember there are plenty of other choices available that may better suit your family's needs.

In summary, finding the right general practitioner to care for a child with sickle cell disease is crucial for addressing their medical, emotional, and psychological needs. A good GP will be caring, knowledgeable, and proactive in collaborating with specialists. By considering factors such as experience, communication skills, availability, and willingness to work with other healthcare providers as part of your child's care team, you can find providers who will support and improve your child's health as they live with this condition.

17

Understanding Haematologists

Seeking help from a haematologist who specialises in sickle cell disease is crucial for managing this complex, lifelong condition. Haematologists are doctors who diagnose, treat, and manage blood disorders. A haematologist knowledgeable about SCD has significant experience in recognising the disease's complications, is familiar with all treatment options, and can offer a comprehensive approach to care. Here's how to get the right help from a haematologist specialising in SCD:

A haematologist with a specialty in sickle cell disease will have been trained to cover every aspect of the disease. These include care for:

- Diagnosis and Monitoring of Sickle Cell Disease: Blood tests are used to diagnose sickle cell disease, and it is an ongoing requirement to check. For example, haematologists may monitor the proportion of normal red blood cells versus those with an abnormal shape, as well as look for any signs indicating complications, such as organ damage or anemia.

- Pain Management for Pain Crises: Patients with sickle cell crises will suffer episodes of pain that need to be managed professionally. The specialist can suggest effective strategies for dealing with these crises, as well as offer medications, therapies, and physical treatments, among others.

- Prevention and Treatment of Complications: People suffering from SCD are at risk of complications such as stroke or organ damage, including that to the liver, kidneys, and spleen, which has always accompanied haemophiliacs. Haematologists work hard to detect issues early and provide treatment for them.

- Coordinating with other Specialty Physicians: Sickle Cell Disease is typically treated by a multi-disciplinary team including experts in pain management, psychologists,   orthopaedic specialists, cardiologists, or other physicians far removed from the haematologist's area of expertise. It is the haematologist who forms the core group for this combined approach to patient care, ensuring that each aspect of a patient's health is looked after individually in balance with all others.

1. Finding a Haematologist Specialised in Sickle Cell Disease

When treating Sickle cell disease, it is essential to select a haematologist with experience in treating that condition. The specialty requires special expertise and care. Here's where you can look for your specialist:

- Experience With Sickle Cell Disease: Make sure the haematologist has specific training in the treatment of SCD, including knowledge of new research, treatments, and management techniques. It is also important that they are aware of both paediatric and adult care for patients with sickle cell disease, as needs can change as people grow older.

- Referrals: Ask your family doctor, general practitioner, or paediatrician to refer you to a haematologist who specialises in sickle cell disease. Hospitals or medical clinics with dedicated clinics for treating sickle cell disease may also recommend their own specialists.

- Sickle Cell Centers of Excellence: Look for hospitals or medical centres with experience treating sickle cell disease. Many cities now have centres of excellence specialising in SCD care, which typically include a team including haematologists, nurses, and other specialists focused on sickle cell disease.

- A Patient-Centred Approach: Choose a haematologist who takes a patient- centred, whole-person approach, emphasising not only medical treatments but also emotional support and quality of life. They should be fully inclusive of the patient and family in treatment decisions and clearly explain every possibility in this way.

- Ability To Coordinate Care: A specialised haematologist should be capable of working with other health care practitioners such as pain management specialists, psychologists, orthopaedic surgeons, social workers, etc., to provide comprehensive treatment.

- Accessibility: It is essential that the consultant haematologist is available on call when the need arises.

- Approach to Pain Management: The consultant haematologist must have a solid orientation for taking care of pain in the disease. This may encompass pharmacotherapy alone or pharmacotherapy combined with other forms of medical treatment, as well as referring patients who require specialized care to pain consultants, depending on the circumstances.

- Information About Clinical Trials and New Treatments: Treatments for sickle cell disease are evolving, with new therapies and clinical trials emerging frequently.

- In new treatments for sickle cell disease, a haematologist specialising in SCD must stay up to date. They should be aware of how genes can be manipulated, including hydroxyurea as one of many chemotherapeutic agents now available, blood transfusions, which still require the use of breathing tubes, and bone marrow transplants. Then they can discuss these treatments with you.

- Support Groups and Advocacy Organisations: There are many national or local sickle cell disease organisations, such as Australian Sickle Cell Advocacy Inc., that can provide lists of health care practitioners specialising in SCD. Support groups often recommend doctors based on their own experiences.

- Online Directories: Websites such as the Haematology Society of Australia and New Zealand, American Society of Hematology (ASH), or local medical boards can frequently provide lists of qualified haematologists who specialise in blood diseases.

2.   What to Expect When You Visit Your Haematologist

A visit to a haematologist with appropriate expertise in the disease, sickle cell anaemia, may involve several elements:

- Thorough Medical History: The haematologist may inquire about the child's or patient's personal illness history, family history of sickle cell disease, symptoms, and prior treatments. You should also be prepared to discuss any previous hospitalizations, pain crises ('in crisis'), or other conditions related to sickle cell disease.

- Physical Exam: A physical examination to check for complicating factors may be required if your doctor suspects your signs are suspicious. They might specifically look for signs of illness related to spleen and liver enlargement in sickle cell disease as well as signs of infection and poor growth in children.

- Lab Work and Testing: The haematologist will probably order blood tests to ascertain the amount and size of red blood cells in your system, watch for anaemia critically, and without showing any other signs of infection. Additional diagnostic checks will also be performed, including imaging studies to monitor for stroke or organ damage.

- Extent of Medical Care:The haematologist will develop an individualized treatment plan based on results from examinations and tests. This may include strategies for pain management, adjustments to hydroxyurea dosage, blood transfusions, or referrals to specialists in areas such as pain management or psychology. Any questions?

- Instruction and Support: Expect your haematologist to provide counseling on managing sickle cell disease, including guidance on avoiding triggers for sickling episodes, staying hydrated, choosing the best foods for patients, and the timing of vaccinations for children. The doctor should also inform you about available local resources such as online chat rooms and community support groups that can offer additional support.

3.   Haematologist Care Plans

Once you have established care with a hematology specialist, it is essential to maintain regular communication and collaboration for the long-term management of the disease. Some key points to remember are:

- Regular Follow-Ups: Sickle cell disease requires ongoing monitoring. Regular follow-up visits will help identify changes in the condition, prevent complications, and modify treatment plans as needed.

- Emergency Plan: If a pain crisis occurs or there is another type of emergency related to sickle cell disease, it is essential to have a clear emergency plan in place. A discussion will be held on managing crises, when to seek immediate medical attention, and how to manage pain at home.

- Preventive Care: Work with a haematologist on a preventive care plan that includes vaccinations, routine screenings (such as for stroke risk), and lifestyle adjustments to minimize complications.

- Mental Health Support: Ensure the haematologist understands the emotional and psychological challenges of living with a chronic condition, such as sickle cell disease. They should be able to refer to mental health specialists or provide guidance on managing stress, anxiety, and depression.

- Staying Informed about New Treatments: Sickle cell disease research is ongoing, and new treatments, such as gene therapy and innovative medications, are emerging. Check into what options the haematologist recommends for your child or loved one in terms of any new treatment possibilities or clinical trials.

For managing this chronic condition, meeting with a haematologist who specializes in sickle cell disease is essential. An educated and caring haematologist will provide tailored healthcare, coordinate with other specialists as needed during the initial treatment periods, and keep you informed about the latest treatments and developments in sickle cell hematology. By consulting a haematologist with specialized knowledge about sickle cell disease, you can help ensure the best possible care for your child or loved one and prevent complications that may arise as a result of their condition.

Regular checks and childhood screenings for sickle cell disease (SCD) are crucial for managing lifelong conditions and preventing potential complications. Regular checks are essential for monitoring one's health, identifying emerging issues early, and adjusting medication dosage as necessary. Everyone who visits with the doctor helps ensure that a patient with sickle-cell disease receives all the required care and remains in the best of health.

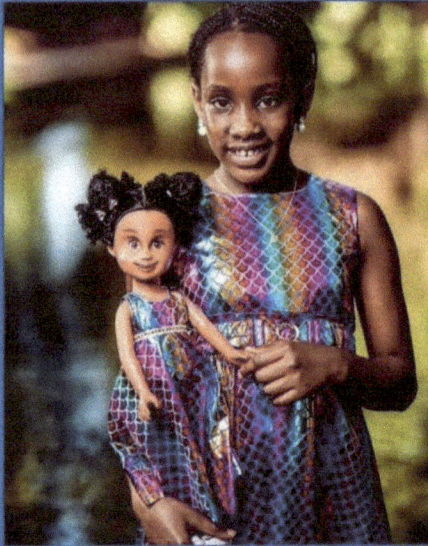
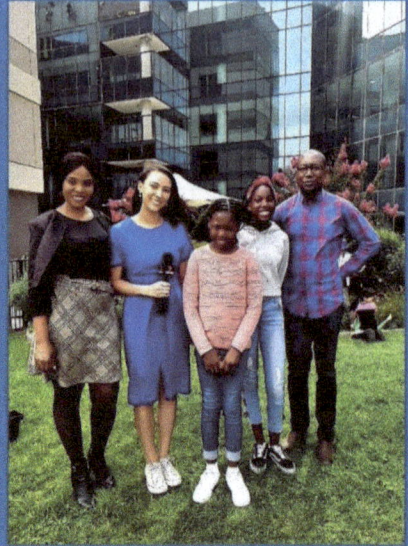
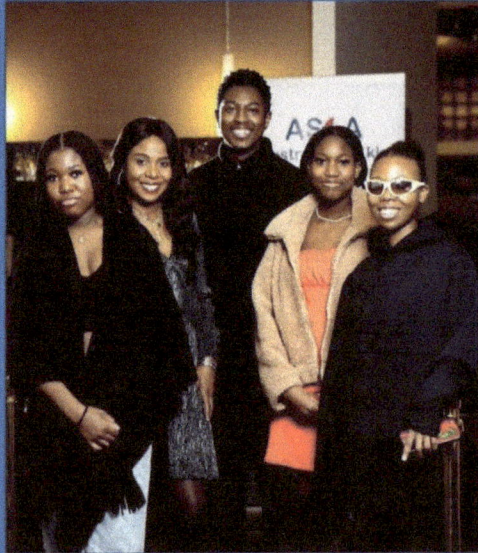

18

Mother's Mental Health Well-being

Caring for a child with sickle cell disease is one of the most difficult and taxing journeys a mother could ever face. However, it is also gratifying. This road is filled with love, sacrifice, uncertainty, and measures that might need to be included. While caring for your child quickly becomes the most significant concern, it's also essential to prioritize your mental and emotional well-being. Where the path of caregiving takes a toll not only on the body but also on the mind and spirit, it is easy to forget that mental health exhaustion, anxiety, and feelings of isolation will follow like a shadow everywhere you go.

Glancing back during those early days after my daughter was diagnosed, I found myself submerged in an emotional flood. Fear was probably the most familiar thing I knew. Fear for her life as another sickle cell crisis occurred; fear of hospital admissions; fear for the future, and whether unforeseeable events might happen to threaten safety and well- being.

This fear never entirely deserted me, but it changed as my learning increased about the nature of this disease. Alongside fear was an inconsistency of hope and despair. I wanted to believe that treatments such as hydroxyurea or even getting a bone marrow transplant might make an enormous difference to her life. At the same time, however, there was my own sense of despair whenever problems kept cropping up and treatment seemed unrelenting.

Living with these emotions was no less an emotional rollercoaster for which there appeared to be no end. Some days brought relief and new hope; others were bleak and filled with sorrow. Remember that such mood swings are normal and understandable and are not a sign of failure. The journey itself is not linear, and feeling overwhelmed at times is a sign that you need human help.

Physical requirements in this work gave me another reason for carrying a mental and emotional burden. It was a burden usually lightened when I started my day at home for work on my memoirs, where most domestic and household chores awaited me. If you have no other symptoms but any stress, and uninformed self-diagnosis and treatment, permanently altering your state of mind into a self-confessed nervous wreck, that is unacceptable.

The fatigue was profound, and sometimes it wasn't simply a question of needing rest. It was a type of exhaustion that gets into one's very bones, clogging the thinking of people around you, and all work you attempt seems ever more daunting. This weariness is harmful to mental health. It makes it hard to maintain your temper and strength when dealing with difficult children like these. When you seem confused, surely, it's only a matter of time before patience snaps.

It is important to recognise the symptoms that signal a decline in your mental health. For me, once these signs became very clear, I reflected on how, even though I occasionally felt so depressed and would go in a corner. Furthermore, there were moments when irritability would surge out of nowhere! But worst of all, during this period, I felt increasingly cut off from friends and family. My thoughts became foggy, my sleep was restless, my appetite changed, and the burden of caregiving felt overwhelming. It took me some time to realise that these signs simply indicated an overwhelmed spirit, not just temporary stress.

One of the most significant challenges for me was overcoming the guilt associated with taking care of myself. Societal and peer pressure meant that every energy and attention was a mother's duty toward her child. Self-care felt wrong. I remember thinking that if I spent any time resting or doing something for myself, that was time away from caring for my daughter. That concept kept me trapped in recurring cycles of depletion and exhaustion.

Over time, I realised that taking care of my mental health was not a luxury but a necessity. If I were overwhelmed and exhausted, I couldn't provide my daughter with the care or emotional support she needed most. Caring for myself made me more effective, calmer, and clearer-minded.

Building a support network is one of the most vital things you can do for your mental health. I understood that caring for a family member isn't something one person has to do alone. I found ways to get support from relatives who could watch my daughter temporarily so I could rest, friends who listened and helped with practical tasks, and medical professionals who understood the emotional toll of caregiving and referred me for counseling.

Meeting and talking with other parents through support groups was especially comforting. Sharing experiences, fears, and burdens with others who understood this journey firsthand made me feel less alone and much more empowered.

The mental health care provided by professionals has also played a vital role in helping me release my burdens. Mental health professionals helped me challenge negative thinking patterns, set practical life goals, and practice self-love. Many hospitals and clinics offer psychosocial services specifically for caregivers, and I encourage all moms on this journey to utilise these resources. There is strength in seeking support.

Looking after oneself is often easier said than done, particularly when there is not enough time and duties seem overwhelming. However, I came to realise that even small practices pursued consistently had a profound impact on my overall well-being. Mindfulness and meditation were life preservers in stormy seas. If I set aside a few moments each day simply to focus on my breathing or follow some guided meditation, my anxiety began to decrease. Purposes could be centred easily in one minute. If just that much was done daily, remembering the baby steps one needed to take to write before their feet began carrying out acts of love, such as walking up and down in response every time they saw a child, for instance, the result would follow: Not only was your book brought into being But just going for a leisurely walk with the fresh air of the sort we breathe under cover from a tree canopy once every few kilometres or so would do wonders for raising the spirits and ensuring that I could concentrate better on looking after myself. Journaling provided me with a valuable outlet for emotions too complex to express verbally. Creative outlets, such as music and art, provided me with a productive way to channel my feelings.

The basics of sleep and food cannot be neglected. Although maintaining regular sleeping and eating patterns was a challenge, whenever our daughter prioritised them, her resilience and vigour both improved. By eating high-quality food, she sustained her physical strength, which in turn provided a solid foundation for her mental health.

For the most stressful moments, whether during a crisis of sickle cell anemia, in the hospital, or other crisis, you need even more intentional strategies. On these days, I developed easy routines to help distract myself from current stresses and the urgent need for relief: deep breath exercises (to ease panic) or stepping out into the fresh air for a short time. I kept a list of relaxing activities, such as listening to my favourite songs or reading a few pages, to quickly restore calm during my day.And most importantly, I had to remember that at times when my baby's crises came on, other people are experiencing them too. I also worked online to distract myself from the hospital environment.

To preserve my energy and protect my own mental health, however, re-evaluating boundaries was one of the hardest lessons. It involved saying no to social events or additional duties when I felt stressed to the point of exhaustion. It meant speaking openly with family and friends about what I could manage. Although unpleasant at first, boundaries helped conserve my energy. With this method, others also learned to respect and support my limitations.

I found that research on learning to care for someone other than my own child could have nourished my spirit. Caregiving for my daughter is the focus of my life, but being a part of advocacy work and supporting other parents gave me a sense of belonging and hope. Small or large, marking my daughter's growth milestones reminded me of the light travelled. I spent much of my time and energy in search of passion, which went into four places: recreation, schooling, or deepening involvement with society. In this way, what happened to my child could become the most important note on our collective keyboard. It was at this point that, from the point of need, we started chanting, "Mommy?"

For many mothers, me included, spirituality provided an extra sense of peace and calm in their lives. Whether it takes the form of prayer, meditation, or connecting with faith communities, nurturing and maintaining our spiritual health will bring hope to help sustain us through hard times. I encourage all mothers to find such practices, embrace them, and make the ones you adopt work for you personally, rather than just borrowing somebody else's idea without understanding what it means or why it is so potently successful, because they are not trying hard enough!

The fourth pillar of my support system was open communication. Talking frankly and openly with my partner, relatives, and closest friends about the fears I had and what I needed to offload some mental baggage helped them understand how to help me and formed stronger emotional bonds. Sometimes, being able to speak out was its own form of healing.

Celebrating small victories became a necessary part of life. Finding a small moment of reprieve, finally achieving a successful treatment, or simply getting through one day without a crisis helped sustain hope. I adopted practices of gratitude, for example, listing three things that I was thankful for every day. This changed my focus from something challenging that I had to do now or would be difficult tomorrow to being able to look forward with some hope.

Living with a chronic illness means you need to strike a delicate balance between hope for the future and making peace with the present. Although I was doing just that, planning for treatments or cures, I came away from it another person. This practice helped me settle anxieties and find great joy in life's little things.

Listen up, mothers with children suffering from sickle cell disease: You carry the weight of history, yet your mental health remains vulnerable to questioning. You won't find fulfillment until you begin a process of renewing yourself, even if it doesn't seem very different; this may be crucial for both you and future generations. I depend on others' help at every moment!

Even alone, every minute you see is like an eternity. When the path becomes uneven, it isn't good. Seek help, be kind to yourself, and remember that self-care strengthens your ability to care for your child. I was trying to care for my daughter and look out after myself; in the end, fulfilling that one goal helped me be present, hopeful, and resilient. It was a rescue in a stormy sea.

A Practical Mental Health Resource Guide for Caregivers

This guide is divided into four major sections:

1. Daily Self-Care Practices
2. Community Networks and Support Systems
3. Professional Help Resources
4. Mental Health Emergencies

1. Daily Self-Care Practices

These small, simple practices help prevent burnout and nurture daily emotional well- being.

Morning Grounding Routine (5–15 minutes)

- Breathing: Inhale for four counts, hold for four, exhale for six. Repeat 3–5 times.
- Positive Intention: Speak out loud a single sentence, such as *I will do the best I can today* or *Today I am giving myself grace.*
- Check-in One's Physical and Emotional State: Ask yourself, how do I feel now physically and emotionally at this moment? And remember, no critical attitude, just mindfulness.

Daily Self-Compassion

- Affirmations: Keep in your mirror a sticky note with an empowering affirmation, such as I am a caring and capable mother.
- I deserve peace and kindness.
- Doubt all you want; I will stand here as long as it takes. I refuse to take another 10,000 steps (which in Japan were measured with feet—10 feet per half-length—adding up to 30 yards). Next year, I'll be scolded for a lesson.
- Reduce Your Guilt: Whenever you feel stressed and need to take a break, or ask for help from others, don't forget to say to yourself: "This is not selfish, it's self- preservation."
- Short Breaks (10 minutes)
- Step outside and take a deep breath of fresh air.
- Drink tea or water with attention, feel the warmth over your tongue or the coolness in your mouth.
- Do simple stretches.
- Listen to a calming playlist.

Sleep and Nutrition

- Try to nap when your child takes a nap or has a break. It doesn't have to be for a long time; even 20-30 minutes will restore your spirits.
- Keep nuts, fruits, and smoothies handy.
- Drink plenty of water—tiredness often arises from dehydration.

2. Community or Social Connections:

A lone person soon falls sick. Being part of a group is beneficial for one's health.

Parent Support Groups

- Online: Join groups on Facebook and WhatsApp that focus on parenting with SCD.
- At Local Hospitals: Many general hospitals have parent meetups or programs for peer support.

Respite Care

For some "time out," contact relevant local carers' organisations (e.g., Carer Gateway Australia).

Faith and Cultural Community

- Contact spiritual or cultural associations for prayer, meditation, all kinds of nourishment. Emotional care should be sought from them also.
- In practical ways, we need the help of trusted members. Can they take care of our children? Do the work of the kitchen? Or help us run errands?

3. Professional Help Network: When to Seek Help

- Prolonged sadness, anger, or numbness
- Sleep is a problem, not just your child's care
- Hope is waning, overwhelmed by isolation
- Unable to function in daily life

Where To Find Mental Health Support

- General Practitioner (GP): Ask them for a mental health care plan and what hospitals or sickle cell units they can recommend.
- Hospital-based social workers, psychologists, or therapists: Many good hospitals also have someone to help families.
- Community counsellors.
- Australia: Beyond Blue, PANDA, Carers Australia, SANE Australia, International: Mental Health America, Better Help, Talk Space, Low-Cost and No-Charge Counselling Services, University clinics with students volunteering as psychologists under supervision by their professors

- Community Health Centers
- Voluntary organizations assisting family members who suffer from chronic illness
- Australian Sickle Cell Advocacy Inc 1300 148 124

4. **Mental Health Emergencies**

Sometimes you get to the end of your tether. It has to be prepared for, and as far as possible, for those moments of crisis.

In Case of a Crisis (example: Australia—please customise to your country)

- Telephone lifeline: 13 11 14

- Beyond Blue Support Service: 1300 22 4636

- Parent line: 1300 30 1300

- Mental Health Emergency Response Line (MHERL): 1800 676 822

Crisis Coping Plan

Take this plan in writing (on a piece of paper, a note in your phone):

- People you can call or text
- The Ames technique to calm yourself down. Note: The Ames technique, first set out in Training, and which Mao T sees in the next edition of Quarterly Management How-to Manual (Chien I-chiait 1992), was once more to call forth protest from the parents who said, "But we don't have the money. If we are lucky, we can barely afford our food for every day and don't ask where we should get this extra RMB 800 to buy books." That's true, but then, too, all parents do it just this way

- 1 positive affirming statement (e.g., "This moment will pass.")

- Where is the nearest walk-in or emergency care facility?
- Exercise for the Reflection of Mums

These are activities a mother can do on a weekly or monthly basis to improve emotional clarity and radiance.

Reflection 1: Emotional Inventory

Prompt:

What is the dominant feeling in me today? Where do I feel this in my body?

What is the content of this feeling in terms of meaning?

Pray, let us take counsel on behalf of our mother, who is now living on the mainland under so much pressure and who must endure loneliness, pain, and sheer human existence without respite from those who would seek her out for marriage purposes.

Purpose: To help mothers with their feelings. Who doesn't know that being healthy and flourishing is the most important thing?

In A Short Talk about Prosperity, Providing. Your Future Happiness, and Whether or Not You Are Healthy, Mastering the Basic Laws of Human Life That Will Improve Your Fate - Chapter 4 060 Doctor of Mine. If you feel that something has not gone as planned or thought through, phone a technician. Do they offer such service in the U.S. market, we wonder?

Reflection 2: Letter to Myself

Instructions

- Imagine that you are talking to yourself as a best friend and write a short letter.
- No matter what's happening to you, something interesting is happening inside you.
- Pity yourself for your suffering.
- Wishing you well and loving kindness always

For the record, this sort of thing strengthens the assistance you give yourself, adds self- compassion, and confirms that you ARE worthy of love.

Reflection 3: What Gave Me Strength This Week?

Prompt:

- Can you remember one moment this week when you felt successful or strong? Please tell us about it!
- How did you come out ahead at that moment?
- How can you extend that experience further into the future?

Purpose: Increases resilience, highlights coping tools that we are already using.

Reflection 4: Release the Guilt

Prompt:

- What is something, in your capacity as a parent, that you are feeling guilty about?
- Write a reply from the perspective of a mommy who is sympathetic and understanding.
- What would you tell a friend in the same situation?

Purpose: Changes the people's power of negative self-talk and is conducive to emotions

Reflection 5: Values and Vision

Prompt:

- What kind of mother do I want to be (not perfect, but present)?
- What is the most important thing I hope to impress upon my child?
- For me, what is "good day?"

Purpose: Centers you back on what really matters and sets intentional parenting goals

Reflection 6: Joy and Gratitude Collage

Prompt:

- List (or draw) 5 things that brought you joy in the last month.
- These things could be big or small joys–smiles, milestones, laughter, or peace.

Add to that three things that you are thankful for right now.

Purpose: Illuminates sombre days and encourages changes in viewpoint

Reflection 7: If I Had One Day Only for Me...

Prompt:

- What would constitute a successful, satisfying day of self-care, leisure, and joy for you?

- What small steps might you take during your week, even in little ways, so that you can give yourself something efficiently?

Purpose: Promotes imagining the future with balance and purposeful consideration for what we can achieve

Final Encouragement

You are not just a caregiver, you are a person too, and you deserve health, happiness, and wholeness. You don't have to wait for a crisis to start taking care of your mental health. Begin today, lovingly and in little ways. Let this be your gentle companion, an island of peace, a message that your wellbeing is special, and you matter very much.

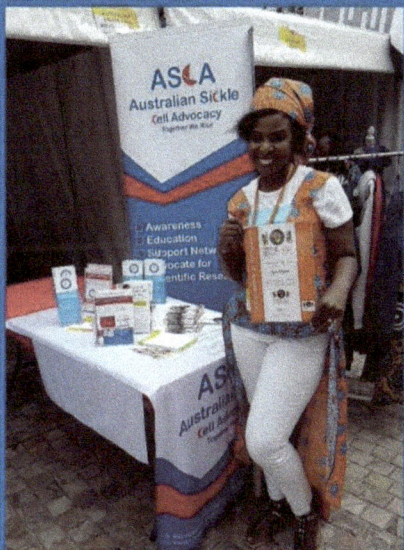

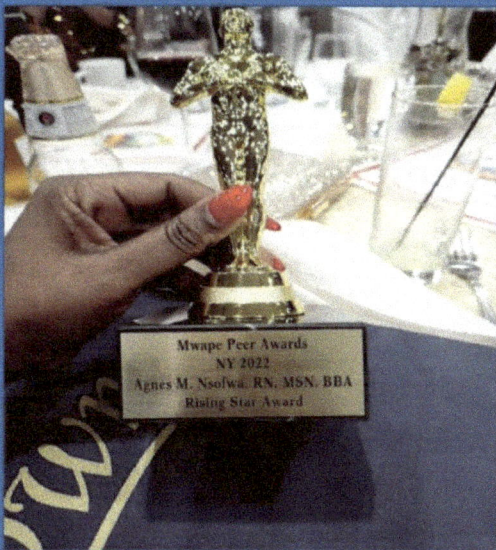

Mwape Peer Awards
NY 2022
Agnes M. Nsofwa, RN, MSN, BBA
Rising Star Award

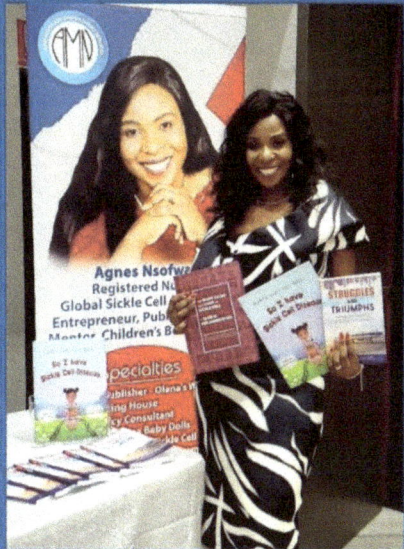

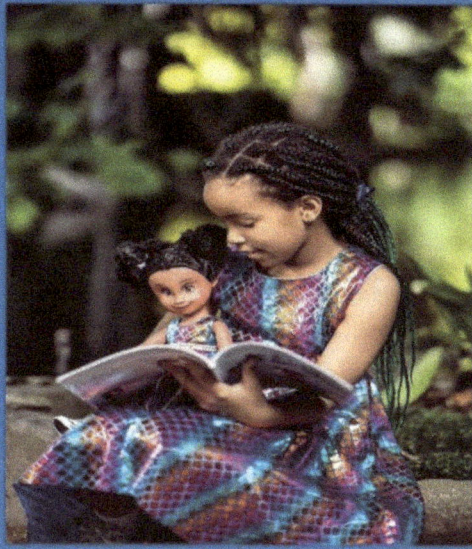

The End of a Journey—And the New Road Ahead

When I reflect on everything that has happened, I feel grateful, humble, hopeful, and determined. This book of mine has taken us from the shock of diagnosis through treatment, the small successes, the occasional huge failures, and then on to further work: increasing awareness and strengthening support networks. This journey has changed me. I hope it has affected you too.

1. From Diagnosis to Advocacy

At the heart of this tale is a mother's care. It is fierce, unwavering, made in hospital rooms and corridors, in whispers with specialists, and in the nightly agony as well as small victories unreported. In recording the story of this journey, my intention has been to demonstrate how love can become a form of activism and how, in caring for a child with a chronic illness, parents become doctors, advocates, professors, and the people who make history. Out of this transformation, real change will follow.

We started in fear and doubt. We were not familiar with this illness. We did not know why crises arose, and certainly, we didn't know the kind of complicated health-care system we would be up against. But one day is just another day added to the count of weeks in a month; admissions add appointments, and it's all about learning. We ask questions. We connect the dots. Now, with this growing carpet of information, we have action: training teachers on how to handle schools; bands of mothers taking families under their wings; getting healthcare professionals to listen and understand—and building a voice that will be heard far beyond any hospital ward.

2.   A Community of Strength

Notably, our discoveries highlight the robustness that arises from unity. No one should have to endure sickle cell disease alone. Telling our story to audiences at the playground and the fair, on social media and in schoolrooms, in the doctor's office and at policy forums, we write stories, and it has had an impact. It has been very powerful. It has touched people's hearts because every parent shares the same hope, and every oppressed community deserves to have its story told.

For us, World Sickle Cell Day, the Food Festival, and the school workshops are not simply campaigns of awareness. These events are lifelines. This is where children and families will also see themselves, the real-life blood society can draw on, people with blood disorders; at last, this is where nurses and doctors can feel firsthand how students' ignorance turns toward compassion. This is where stigma begins to open its door and understanding—and inclusion—take their place in society.

3.   Changing the Record

A story has the power, when it unfolds, to shape narratives and change the record. When a distracted teacher hears "fatigue" instead of "laziness," when an awareness of the early signs of crisis becomes routine for doctors because they are trained to spot the, when 'the watchers' see life, when children and their families at last feel recognized rather than forgotten, these are the results of awareness rooted in lived experience.

The numbers matter. The stories matter more. We couple instruction with empathy. When we appeal to politicians for their support in brief snippets of testimony, at school gates, and in warm conversations via social media, we do more than ask for money or regulation; we ask for people's recognition. We say, "See us. Understand us. Walk this road together with us!"

And very slowly, sometimes grudgingly, reactions come. We have received updated resources and regulations, and policies have been developed with students with sickle cell disease in mind. Money has begun to pour into both scientific research and outreach efforts aimed at educating the public about sickle cell anemia, its origins, and potential cures. These are small wins, though they are real and substantial. They remind us that changes may take a very long time but are intractable all the same.

4.   A Mother's Hope

If there's one thing I hope to share, it's this: no other mother or father will ever feel as isolated and alone as we did during those first nights in intensive care. No parent should have to struggle to understand what teachers are saying or what hospital protocols require. No child should be made to stand still at recess because their friends do not recognize that they are in pain.

We need the voices of families, the ears of schools, a changing health system, and the involvement of neighbourhoods. We need research to seek cures and therapies to ward off crises. We need cultural competency in healthcare, policies that represent diverse perspectives, and early, clear genetic education so that parents are informed from the outset about the choices available to them.

5.   Hope Every Day

However, amid a crisis, people still find beauty. I saw it in my daughter's strength, facing aching bones and tired limbs with greater determination than mine. I saw it in teachers who watch for signs and say, "You needn't rush." I saw it in the community that wept when it saw the tiny information stall, then showed signs of life again. I saw it in health teams that learn how to do things differently, and whose work shows respect. I saw it in parents who help each other out.

These are not big blessings. But they are the kernel of hope and healing. They are the building blocks of community. And they make me believe that the future, though strewn with difficulties, will still be better.

6.   What Comes Next

There is still so much work to be done. For instance, we need to have:

- Expanded support in rural, remote, and underserved areas so that no families are beyond the pale
- Multilingual and culturally tailored educational resources for families with low incomes, so that nothing keeps them in the dark
- Partnerships with other multicultural societies that have their own comprehension and history of health inequity, which can enrich the discussion
- Policy lobbying, maintaining the investment in research (subsidised treatment programs are called for; bring new treatment options into Australia and have them included in national health strategies)
- Financial support when we find partner organisations
- Greater awareness and support services for schools, so that each child may learn and grow in society free from the feeling that they are "different"
- Not just focusing on life span, but quality of life, mental health, pain management, and long-term organ health in clinical trials of disease treatments.

7.   Leading the Light Forward

This book ends with the close of this chapter, but its journey does not end. I want to invite you to take up the torch that we have lit. If you are a parent, speak out and tell your child's story. If you're a teacher, stay open. If you're a health care worker, listen to the news and remember the person behind the pulse. If you're a policymaker, remember that these lives go beyond statistics. Stand with people in the community, ask questions, show empathy, and be there for those families that need it most. If we reach out and touch one another, we will be a community moving forward into the future.

Care gives rise to care, and all the minor matters above are great events. Every conversation, every training session, every charity it all counts.

Final Words

Taking care of a child living with sickle cell disease has taught me profoundly: It is the weakest who have the most challenging quest of vulnerability who bring strength. We reach out to others, and they respond. When we tell our stories, people listen. And as communities are built, there is hope for change.

Today, as we bring this book together, we don't say goodbye. Instead, we say go forward. Go forward to schools where they have invisible disabilities. Go forward to clinics where children are treated well, and women are sometimes included. Go forward toward the day when policies protect ALL families. Go forward until conversation causes change!

The journey continues, as one child wins a day more, one family finds its voice, and a community says to us: "We see you for who you truly are, now completely and everything this entitles you."

Thank you for joining us on this walk. Together, however, we are providing not just the care of an individual with a lifetime of sickle-cell disease, but also reciprocally strengthening society. We are building a tomorrow in which all straits are not silent and no one's future hangs quietly unnoticed.

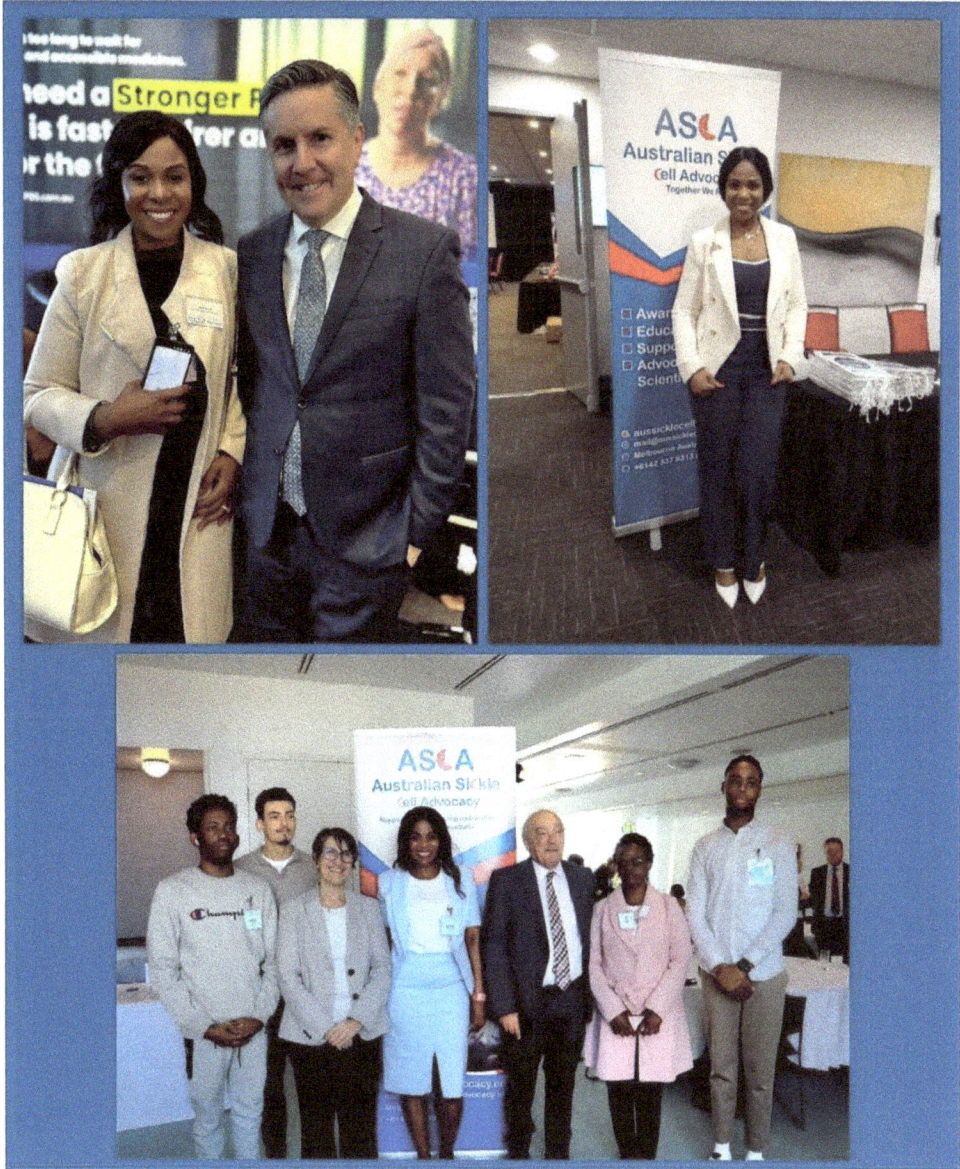

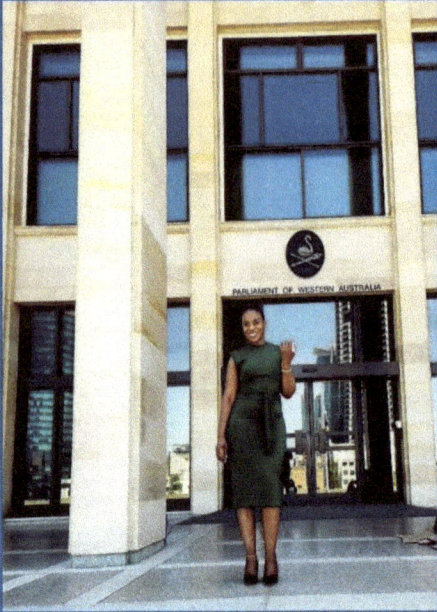

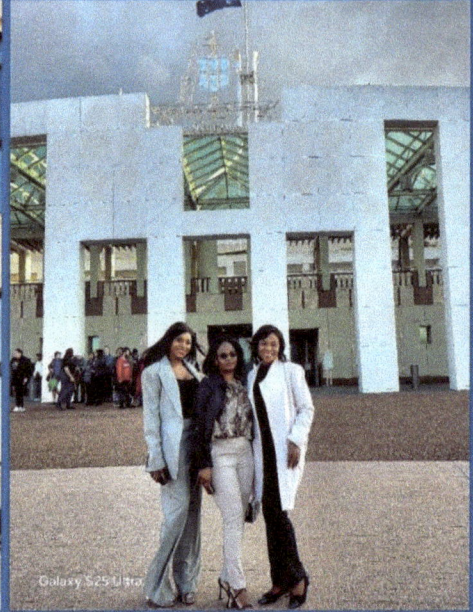

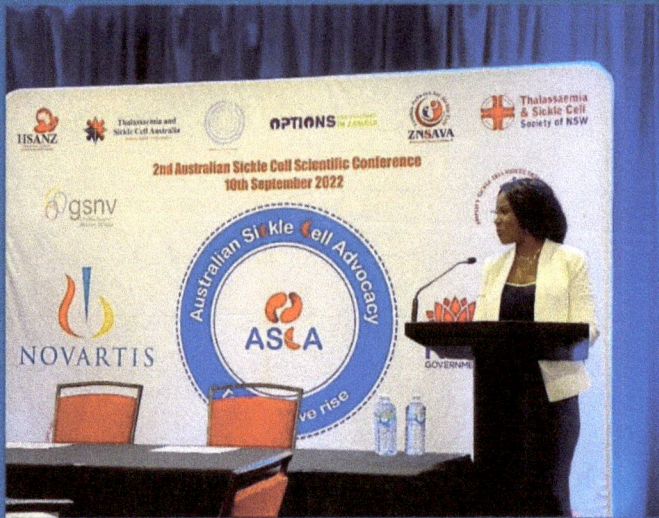

Appendix 1: Understanding Routine Blood Tests and Vital Signs (Caregiver Handout)

Vital Signs—What to Watch For

Vital Sign	Normal Range (Child)	What It Tells You
Temperature	36.5°C-37.5°C	Fever may signal infection or crisis
Heart Rate	70-120 bpm	Increased with pain, fever, or anemia
Respiratory Rate	20-30 breaths/min	Increased in acute chest or pain
Blood Pressure	Varies by age/size	High = stroke risk; Low = dehydration
Oxygen Saturation	95%-100%	<92% may signal acute chest syndrome

Appendix 2:
Key Blood Tests for Sickle Cell Patients

Test Name	Normal Range / Target	What It Means for Sickle Cell Disease
Haemoglobin (Haemoglobin)	11–13 g/d L (children)	Often lower (6–10); drop may mean a crisis
Reticulocyte Count	0.5%-1.5%	High = marrow is active; low = marrow not responding
White Blood Cells	4,000-11,000/µL	High may suggest infection or inflammation
Platelets	150,000-450,000/µL	May increase after crisis or drop in serious illness
LDH	<280 U/L	High in haemolysis (cell breakdown)
Ferritin	20–300 ng/mL	High in transfusion-related iron overload
Bilirubin	0.1-1.2 mg/dL	High = red cell breakdown, jaundice

- Haemoglobin F% (via electrophoresis): Aim to increase with hydroxyurea.
- Ferritin/Iron: Check with transfusions to avoid overload.

VITAL SIGNS QUICK LOOK

- **SpO$_2$ < 92%?** Get medical help.
- **Fever > 38.5°C?** Emergency until proven otherwise

Appendix 3: Test Frequency Chart by Age

Test / Monitoring	0-2 years	2-10 years	10+ years	On Hydroxyurea	On Regular Transfusions
CBC + Reticulocyte Count	Monthly	Every 2-3 months	Every 3 months	Monthly (initially)	Monthly
Haemoglobin Electrophoresis	Yearly	Yearly	Yearly	2-3x per year	Every 3 months
Liver + Kidney Function (U&E, LFT)	Every 6 months	Every 6 months	Every 3-6 months	Every 3 months	Every 3 months
Ferritin + Iron Studies	Only if transfused	If transfused	Yearly if transfused	Not required routinely	Every 3 months
Transcranial Doppler (TCD)	Not required	Yearly (age 2-16)	Not required after 16	Not affected	Every 6-12 months if at risk
Echocardiogram	Baseline if needed	Every 1-2 years	Every 1-2 years	Every 2 years	Yearly
Urinalysis + Protein	Start at age 5	Yearly	Yearly	Yearly	Yearly

Self-Care Workbook for
WORKING PARENTS

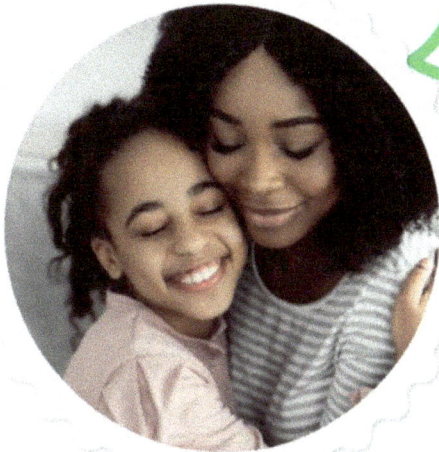

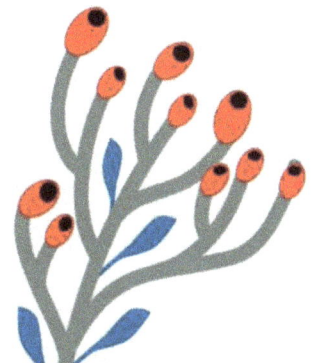

Table of
CONTENTS

- Understanding the meaning of self-care

- Guides to get enough sleep

- Work-life balance

- Self-care habits

- Self-care activity

- Weekly success planner

- Self-care quiz

- Weekly review

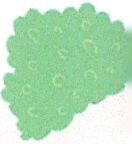

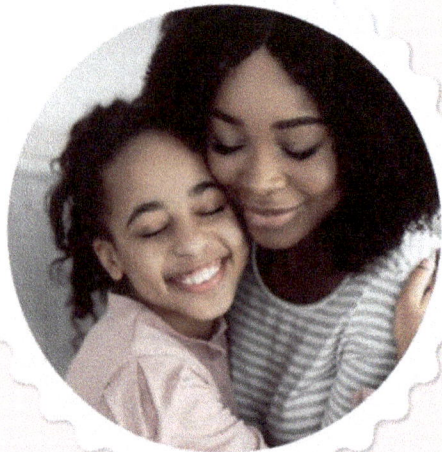

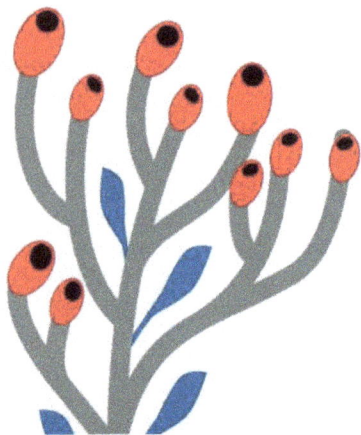

Understanding the Meaning
SELF-CARE

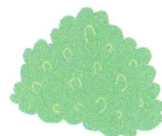

HI MUMS AND DADS,

I hope you're finding the strength to get through each day.
My name is Agnes, and as a mother of a child who has had sickle cell disease, I truly understand the emotional and physical demands that come with this journey.

In this workbook, I'll be sharing practical tips and gentle reminders to help you care for yourself while balancing the responsibilities of parenthood and, for many of us, work or other commitments.

Life as a parent, especially when caring for a child with a chronic condition, can be overwhelming. The constant hospital visits, the sleepless nights, and the worry for your child's wellbeing often leave little room to think about your own needs. Yet, your well-being matters, not just for you, but for your child and family.

This workbook is here to remind you that you are not alone, and that with small, intentional steps, it is possible to care for both your child and yourself.

Best regards,
Agnes MN

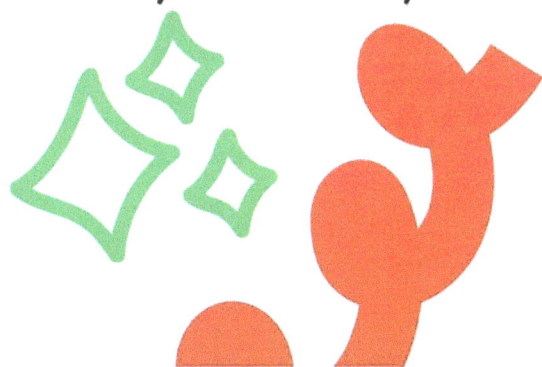

Guides to Get
ENOUGH SLEEP

Working parents can be sleep deprived, you rarely get to shut your eyes or even open your eyes and feel awake. On your maternity leave, all you had to do was taking care of your newborn. It gets worse once you have to return back on track and you're having a hard time maintaining your sleep due to the packed routines. The word give up never exists in parent's dictionary, there are a few hacks you should try to get enough sleep.

As tempted as you may be to stay awake and do things in between your child's bedtime, you should stop the urge to do so. Get some sleep as early as you can, even if it's the time that seems pretty early. You're probably contemplating whether you should sleep or not at those times because you know that you're destined to be awake for several times tonight, but getting some sleep at that early hour helps you to feel refreshed in the next morning.

Getting interrupted sleep is something that you can actually avoid. Rely on your partner, you're not supposed to be taking care of all the burdens by yourself. One of you should create some schedules to be the one to get ready for the midnight wake-ups, you can do three nights on and off in relay with your partner.

If your exhaustion is extremely hard to cope or even disturbs your work performance, consider taking a day off to get the rest that you need and relax. Even if you feel uncomfortable to talk about it with your manager, you should let them know and find the best way to deliver your words.

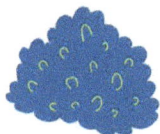

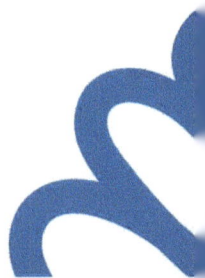

Work-Life Balance
HACKS

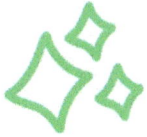

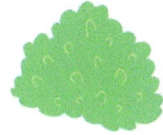

As a working parent, your entire life feels like a balancing act most of the time. You're wiping the milk off your shirt as you're preparing your kids in the morning before you start a tough day at work. It may seems impossible for working parents to find balance in living, but in fact, there are a few things you should consider to do in order to get the work-life balance that you want.

Use time saving ways to do things. Time is precious, especially when you're a working mom, find the shortcuts to the daily activity that you're doing to save some times.

Find a daycare that you trust. Take your time to get your kid the best quality nanny or daycare that you can trust.

Communicate well with your manager. Being a busy working mom doesn't mean that you'll be less productive at work, prove them you can maintain both roles as a mom and as a working woman.

Stop wasting time on unnecessary things. Manage your time well so you will not ruin your productivity at work.

Create meaningful activity with your family for once in a while. Enjoy your time with your family by doing something that your family love.

Share housework with your partner so it will reduce the burden on your shoulder. Communicate well with your partner to find the best solution in sharing the houseworks.

Make friends with other working moms so you will know that you are not alone. There are many working moms out there who are living the same routine as you

Self-Care
HABITS

Go out and inhale the fresh air sometimes

Eat healthy foods and make sure to stay hydrated

Learn new skills

Get some treatments at the salon once in a while

Buy yourself your favorite items at the mall

Do some fun activities with your family to feel happy

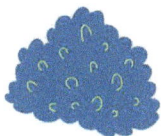 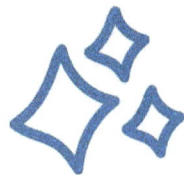

Self-Care

ACTIVITY

Do these activities and write about how they went!

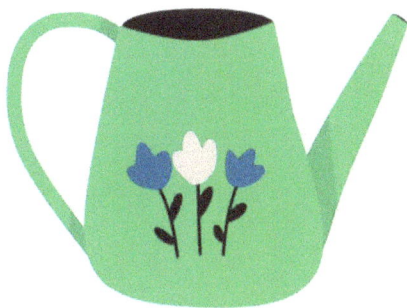

Find a New Hobby

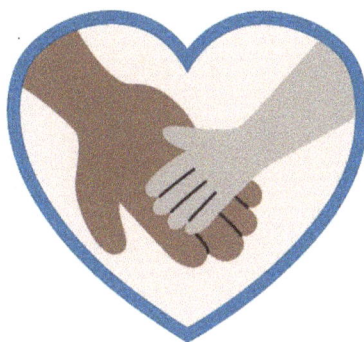

Take Time to Spend
it with Your Family

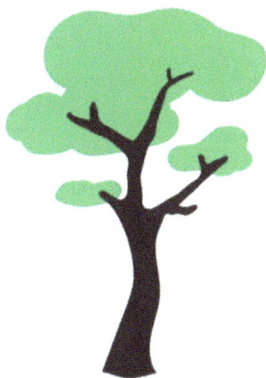

Spend Times in
Nature

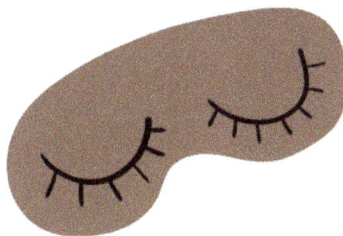

Get 8 Hours
of Sleep

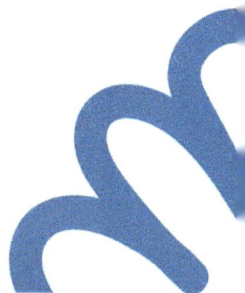

Weekly Success
PLANNER

MY TOP 5 PRIORITIES

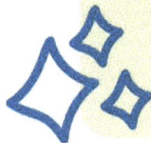

MY TOP 3 GOALS OF THE WEEK

OBSTACLES

SOLUTION TO MY OBSTACLES

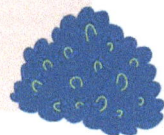

OBSTACLES

I will start _____ next week.
I will start _____ next month.
I will stop _____ next week.
I will stop _____ next month.

Self-Care
QUIZ

Answer the questions with Yes/No and see if you have been taking a good care of yourself through the number of yes in your answers!

I get enough sleep and I feel fresh while working

I eat healthy foods

I spend more times with my family on the weekend

I work well even when I feel tired

I don't find it hard to deal with my routines as a working parent

I take naps

I do all the chores on my own

I always make time for me time

I feel happy and healthy

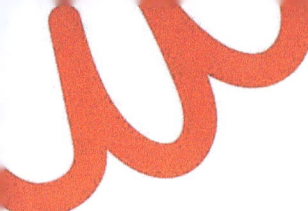
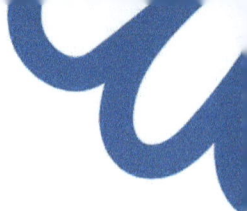

Weekly
REVIEW

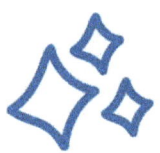
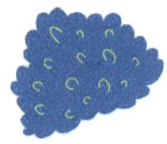

After a week of doing the self-care hacks, write your review below!

WHAT HAVE I ACHIEVED?

WHAT HAVE I LEARNED?

WHAT IS MY FUTURE PLAN AS A WORKING PARENT?

Appendix 4 Self-Care Kits for Caregivers

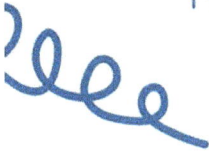

MUM'S SELF CARE

Planner

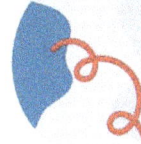

My Mind Goals

- ☐ ....
- ☐ ....
- ☐ ....
- ☐ ....
- ☐ ....
- ☐ ....

Daily Affirmation

My Body Goals

My Note

- --
- --
- --
- --

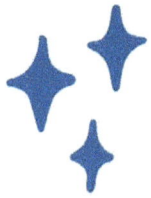

DEAR TO
My future self

Date _____

Dear me,

_____

_____

_____

_____

_____

_____

_____

_____

_____

_____

_____

Signed by,

_____

30 SELF CARE *Challenges*

☐ **01** Cook your favorite meal	☐ **02** Get some sunlight	☐ **03** Watch the sunrise	☐ **04** Practice yoga	☐ **05** Read a book
☐ **06** Write out your goals	☐ **07** Go on a solo date	☐ **08** Drink more water	☐ **09** Take a nice bubble bath	☐ **10** Eat vegetarian meals
☐ **11** Practice gratitude	☐ **12** Organize your closet	☐ **13** Stretch all your muscles	☐ **14** Indulge in your favorite treat	☐ **15** Create your ideal future
☐ **16** Give yourself a manicure	☐ **17** Explore a new city	☐ **18** Go for a walk in nature	☐ **19** Give yourself a facial	☐ **20** Give yourself a break
☐ **21** Watch your favorite movie	☐ **22** Start a new hobby	☐ **23** Drink plenty of water	☐ **24** Make a journal	☐ **25** Watch the sunset
☐ **26** Go to bed earlier	☐ **27** Listen to favorite song	☐ **28** Try a DIY Project	☐ **29** Be gratefull	☐ **30** Learn a new skill

IMPORTANT *Notes*

Date

Other Note

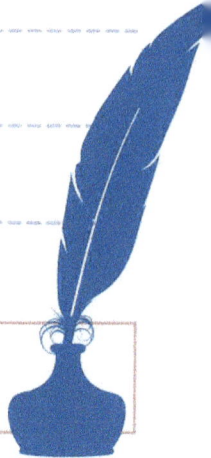

References

1. **American Society of Hematology (ASH). (2020).**
   Sickle Cell Disease Guidelines: Cardiopulmonary and Kidney.
   https://www.hematology.org/education/clinicians/guidelines-and-quality-care/clinical-practice-guidelines/sickle-cell-disease

2. **Australian Sickle Cell Advocacy Inc. (2024).**
   Understanding Blood Tests and Vitals in SCD: Parent & Caregiver Toolkit.
   Internal resource developed for families in Australia.

3. **British Society for Haematology. (2021).**
   Guidelines for the use of hydroxyurea in sickle cell disease.
   https://b-s-h.org.uk/guidelines

4. **Centers for Disease Control and Prevention (CDC). (2022).**
   Complications and Treatments of Sickle Cell Disease.
   Retrieved from https://www.cdc.gov/ncbddd/sicklecell/treatments.html

5. **Kanter, J., & Kruse-Jarres, R. (2013).**
   Management of sickle cell disease from childhood through adulthood.
   Blood Reviews, 27(6), 279–287.
   https://doi.org/10.1016/j.blre.2013.09.001

6. Leger, T., Jacquier, A., Castelli, M., Finance, J., Lagier, J. C., Million, M., Parola, P., Brouqui, P., Raoult, D., Bartoli, A., Gaubert, J. Y., & Habert, P. (2020). Low-dose chest CT for diagnosing and assessing the extent of lung involvement of SARS-CoV-2 pneumonia using a semi quantitative score. PLoS One, 15(11), e0241407.

7. **National Heart, Lung, and Blood Institute (NHLBI). (2014).**
   Evidence-Based Management of Sickle Cell Disease: Expert Panel Report, 2014.
   U.S. Department of Health and Human Services.
   https://www.nhlbi.nih.gov/health-topics/evidence-based-management-sickle-cell-disease

8. **National Institutes of Health (NIH). (n.d.).**
   Sickle Cell Disease—Diagnosis and Management.
   Retrieved from https://www.nhlbi.nih.gov/health/sickle-cell-disease

9. **NICE Guidelines (UK)—National Institute for Health and Care Excellence. (2016).**
   Sickle cell disease: Managing acute painful episodes in hospital.
   https://www.nice.org.uk/guidance/qs58

10. **Royal Children's Hospital Melbourne (RCH). (2023).**
    Sickle Cell Disease Clinical Guidelines.
    https://www.rch.org.au/clinicalguide/guideline_index/Sickle_cell_disease/

11. **Transcranial Doppler Screening for Stroke Prevention in Sickle Cell Anemia. (1998).**
    STOP Trial.
    New England Journal of Medicine, 339, 5–11.
    https://doi.org/10.1056/NEJM199807023390102

12. **Treadwell, M. J., Barreda, F., & Hassell, K. (2016).**
    Self-efficacy and health-related quality of life in adults with sickle cell disease.
    The Journal of the National Medical Association, 108(2), 90–95.
    https://doi.org/10.1016/j.jnma.2016.02.004

13. **Ware, R. E., de Montalembert, M., Tshilolo, L., & Abboud, M. R. (2017).**
    Sickle cell disease.
    The Lancet, 390(10091), 311–323.
    https://doi.org/10.1016/S0140-6736(17)30193-9

14. **Yawn, B. P., Buchanan, G. R., Afenyi-Annan, A. N., et al. (2014).**
    Management of sickle cell disease: Summary of the 2014 evidence-based report by expert panel members.
    JAMA, 312(10), 1033–1048.
    https://doi.org/10.1001/jama.2014.10517

THE END

THANK YOU FOR READING

IF YOU HAVE ANY QUESTIONS CONTACT ME ON

OLANASWORLD@GMAIL.COM

MELBOURNE AUSTRALIA

Agnes MN

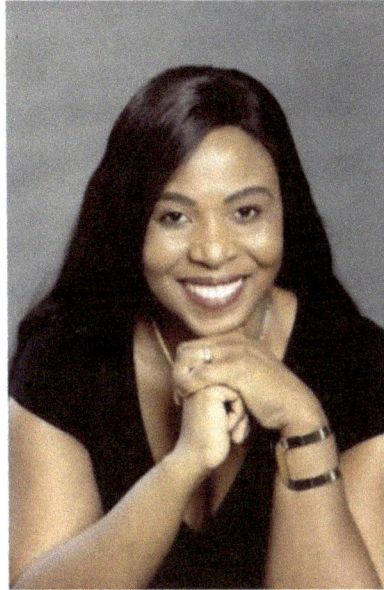

www.ingramcontent.com/pod-product-compliance
Lightning Source LLC
Chambersburg PA
CBHW040927050426
42334CB00062B/3258